The Look You Like

The Look You Like

MEDICAL ANSWERS TO 400 QUESTIONS ON SKIN AND HAIR CARE

LINDA ALLEN SCHOEN
PAUL LAZAR, M.D.

Senior Editor
John S. Strauss, M.D.

Editorial Consultants
D'Anne Kleinsmith, M.D.
James J. Leyden, M.D.
Alan R. Shalita, M.D.

Sponsored by the
American Academy of Dermatology

Marcel Dekker, Inc.   New York and Basel

Library of Congress Cataloging-in-Publication Data

Schoen, Linda Allen.
  The look you like : medical answers to 400 questions on skin and
hair care / Linda Allen Schoen, Paul Lazar.
     p.   cm.
  Includes index.
  ISBN 0-8247-8146-5 (alk. paper)
  1. Skin—Care and hygiene.   2. Hair—Care and hygiene.   3. Beauty,
Personal.   I. Lazar, Paul.   II. Title.
RL87.S343   1989
616.5—dc20

                                                        89-11727
                                                           CIP

Sponsored by the
American Academy of Dermatology
1567 Maple Avenue
Evanston, Illinois 60201

This book is printed on acid-free paper.

MARCEL DEKKER, INC.
270 Madison Avenue, New York, New York 10016

Current printing (last digit):
10 9 8 7 6 5 4 3 2 1

PRINTED IN THE UNITED STATES OF AMERICA

Preface

The Look You Like is designed to answer the numerous questions commonly asked by the public about care of the skin, hair, and nails, as well as cosmetics. The concept of this book derived from the previous publications of the American Medical Association Committee on Cutaneous Health and Cosmetics, *The Look You Like* and *The AMA Book of Skin and Hair Care*. While those books served as a guide, the current book has been totally rewritten and many new chapters have been added by Ms. Linda Allen Schoen and Dr. Paul Lazar. It is published under the auspices of Dermatology Services, Inc., a division of the American Academy of Dermatology, many of whose members have assisted in the editorial and review process. We believe that the question and answer format is unique and specifically designed to respond to the concerns of dermatological patients and the public at large. *The Look You Like* should prove to be of value to consumers, dermatologists, and members of the health care and cosmetic industry.

Alan R. Shalita, M.D.
President, Dermatology Services, Inc.

Acknowledgments

The authors and editors would like to take this opportunity to thank the various scientists and other physicians who so generously gave of their time in reviewing chapters and other portions of the manuscript for this book. Many of their suggestions have been incorporated in the present text. The final responsibility, however, rests with the authors and editors.

Grateful acknowledgement is extended to Myra Barker, Ph.D., Mary Kay Cosmetics, Inc.; Earle Brauer, M.D., Revlon, Inc.; John Corbett, Ph.D., Clairol, Inc.; Richard Gibbs, M.D., NYU Medical Center; Barbara A. Gilchrest, M.D., Boston University; William Jordan, M.D., Medical College of Virginia; Nicholas Pelliccione, Ph.D., Estee Lauder, Inc.; George Pollack, Ph.D., Cosmair, Inc.; Kenzo Sato, M.D., University of Iowa; Richard Scher, M.D., Columbia University; John Voorhees, M.D., University of Michigan; and Charles Zviak, L'Oreál-Lancôme.

The authors also wish to express their deep appreciation to Ms. Kathleen Deakins and Ms. Alene Lain, who assisted in the preparation of the manuscripts, coordinated the various revisions and editorial changes, and distributed the texts to the various editors.

Contents

21. The Sun and Skin   239

22. Acne   253

23. Psoriasis   273

The Look You Like

1

Hair:
Facts and Basic Care

Basic Hair Care

What do I need to know to practice good basic hair care?

The first step in basic hair care is learning something about hair structure.

Hair is an appendage of the epidermis, the outer layer of skin. Hairs are derived from specialized epidermal cells that form the hair follicles (see diagram). Hair follicles develop before birth. The average scalp contains from 80,000 to 120,000 hair follicles. This number is determined genetically, and no new hair follicles form after birth.

The only growing, or live, portion of the hair is the hair root (papilla), found at the base of the follicle. As soon as the cells that make up hair are produced, they die and become cornified (hardened) to form the hair shaft. The hair shaft, like the epidermis, is composed of cells filled with keratin, a protein. The hair shaft is gradually pushed up the follicle tube toward the surface of the scalp at a rate of about ⅓ to ½ inch per month (for more details about hair growth see the following question and answer).

The hair shaft is lubricated with an oily substance (sebum) secreted by the sebaceous (oil) glands that open into the follicle. There's also a muscle attached to each hair follicle (the arrector pili) that can cause hair to "stand on end" or produce "gooseflesh."

The hair is composed of three layers: an inner layer called the medulla (although sometimes the medulla is not present); a middle layer called the cortex, which contains the pigments that pro-

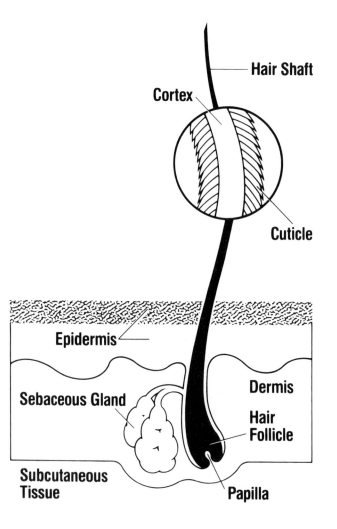

vide hair color; and an outer (covering) layer called the cuticle (see diagram).

The cuticle is composed of overlapping cells (cuticles) that resemble shingles on a roof (see diagram). When the cuticle layer is intact, with the "shingles" flat, the hair feels smooth, doesn't tangle easily, and looks shiny because light bounces off the smooth surface. If the cuticle layer becomes damaged from trauma such as brushing or combing or as a consequence of damage from hair processing for coloring, bleaching, or straightening, some of the cuticular cells begin to separate and may even get torn off. It's as if a tornado hit a shingled roof, lifting some shingles and tearing off others. The surface is now rough and pitted. The hair tangles more easily. It looks dull and drab because light does not bounce evenly off this rough surface. The ends may fray and split into layers (split ends).

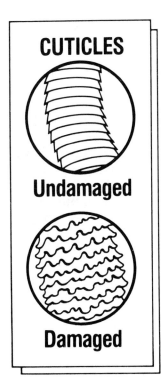

CUTICLES

Undamaged

Damaged

Since the hair shaft is dead, it cannot repair itself. The damage is permanent. To once again have shiny, easy-to-manage hair, you must wait for new, undamaged hair growth to appear. Hair products such as conditioners provide only temporary improvement, but they may help to prevent further damage.

The goal of basic hair care, therefore, is to minimize damage to the cuticle layer. And the byword of all hair care should be *gentle*. Don't *abuse* hair.

Shampoo gently. The hair swells on contact with water and becomes more fragile when it is wet. Wet the hair thoroughly with water that is not too hot. Apply shampoo and work up a good lather. Massage the scalp with the tips of the fingers instead of the fingernails to avoid scalp irritation. If your hair is excessively long or damaged, divide the scalp into quadrants and shampoo each separately. Rinse thoroughly to remove all traces of shampoo residue. If your hair is oily or especially soiled, you may need a second lather to get the hair and scalp thoroughly clean.

If your hair is damaged or dry, use a conditioner following the shampoo. A conditioner will coat the hair shaft with a thin film that smooths down roughened cuticular cells and fills in the roughened, uneven surface. Combing and brushing are easier. Hair doesn't tangle as badly and regains its gloss and luster because light bounces more evenly off this smooth surface.

Wrap your hair in a towel and pat it dry; don't rub the hair or you will rough up the surface of the cuticular layer or even break fragile hair shafts.

Comb wet hair with a wide-toothed, smooth-edged comb with blunt tips (no sharp teeth). Never brush wet hair; it's too elastic and may snap with pulling. Work out tangles by combing gently, starting from the ends and working toward the scalp.

If you use heat-drying or styling appliances, make sure the temperature is not too high. Set the dryer on medium instead of high. It will take longer to dry your hair but you are less apt to cause unnecessary damage. Don't use curling irons and electric curlers on a daily basis. Limit their use to two or three times per week at the most. Use smooth-surfaced or foam rollers instead of brush rollers. Brush your hair no more than is necessary for styling, and use a natural-bristle or nylon brush that has blunt, rounded tips.

Avoid overprocessing by bleaches, tints, or permanent-waving or straightening products. Carefully read and follow directions for home-use products. If your hair is damaged, you should have it done by a professional hairdresser rather than try to do it yourself. The professional knows how to minimize damage.

Protect the hair from the damaging, drying effects of the sun. If you swim, be sure to promptly shampoo your hair to remove chlorine and other chemicals, or salt water, all of which may produce drying.

Hair begins to look shaggy and uneven about a month after a haircut, so regular visits to the hairdresser or barber are a necessary part of good, basic hair care.

Many of these points are discussed in more detail later in this chapter and in Chapters 3–6.

Hair Grows in Cycles

Does hair grow continuously? If so, why can't I grow long hair?

Some animals, such as sheep and poodles, have hair that grows continuously, but human hair does not. It grows in cycles, with a growth phase followed by a resting phase. The length of the growing cycle determines how long your hair will ever grow—assuming you never cut it, of course. And since your growth cycle is determined genetically, there is nothing you can do about it.

The hairs on the scalp have growing cycles that vary from two to six years, during which time the hair grows about ⅓ to ½ inch per month. Then each hair goes into a transitional stage during which it stops growing, develops a clublike tip, and separates from the root (papilla). This hair is then shed. When a new growth cycle is initiated, a new hair is formed. The growth cycles of the hairs of the scalp are out of sequence with one another, so only about 15% of the hairs scattered throughout the scalp are in the resting phase, and thus shed, at any one time. Otherwise we would all develop relative baldness periodically, like some animals.

Because the length of the growing cycle can vary so much, there is also considerable variation in how long different individuals' hair will grow. Only people with an extremely long growing cycle will ever have hair that reaches below the waist. The person with a minimum hair growth cycle can hope for hair only up to about 12 inches long.

Since you are unhappy with the length of your hair, you probably have a shorter growth cycle. To find out if this is the case, check the tips. The tips of normally growing, undamaged, and uncut hairs come to a fine point. If you have normal fine tips your hair is growing as long as it will. If the tips are sharply cut, blunt, or jagged, it means that the shafts have been cut or broken and your hair is not growing to its normal length. The culprit could be excessive heat from electric styling appliances; exposure to sunlight or chlorinated or salt water; or too frequent brushing, over-bleaching, straightening, or other such treatments. If this is the case, proper care will help give you longer hair.

In rare cases, short hair results from a medical problem (e.g., malnutrition, severe hormonal imbalance, improper thyroid functioning). But if you're feeling well and have no specific complaints, this is probably not your problem.

Straight Versus Curly Hair

Some hair is straighter, grows longer, and seems to be different in various ethnic groups. Why does this occur?

The degree of curliness depends on the shape of the hair in cross-section. The rounder the hair, the straighter it is. The more oval or ribbonlike the shape, the curlier the hair. The scalp hair of Orientals is usually straight because it is round in cross-section. Caucasians' scalp hair in cross-section is more slender and elliptical, while blacks' scalp hair is flattened and ribbonlike. Some even have curved hair follicles, which may also affect curliness.

The distribution of hair varies. For instance, as a rule, Caucasians have much more beard, axillary, body, and pubic hair than Orientals do. Wide variations exist because of the years of mixing of the world's ethnic groups.

Hair Color

Why do people have different colored hair naturally?

The color of hair results from the injection of melanin (pigment) by melanocytes into newly formed hair cells. This occurs at the growing end of the hair (papilla) (see diagram on page 2). The melanocytes in hair produce two compounds: a black-brown melanin, like that produced by skin melanocytes, and a red-yellow pigment called pheomelanin. The black-brown melanin produces brown, black, or blond hair, depending on its concentration. The pheomelanin is responsible for red hair. When pigment is deficient, the hair appears white or gray (see Chapter 2 for more information on gray hair).

Do Blonds Have More Hair?

My girlfriend says she has more hair because hers is blonde while mine is red. Is this true?

Your girlfriend is right; she does have more hair. Blonds average about 120,000 scalp hairs, brunettes have about 100,000, and redheads have the fewest, only about 80,000. But you can tell your girlfriend that you have thicker hairs than she does. Blond hairs are thin or fine, while red hairs are thicker and coarser. Thus, if you weighed all the hairs on each of your heads they would weigh about the same.

Regular Haircuts and Trims Are Helpful

Why does everyone tell me I should get my hair cut regularly? I like long hair and don't see any necessity for spending the money.

If you want your hair to look neat and well-groomed, you should have it trimmed regularly, even if you have long hair.

Each hair on the head grows at its own pace, so within a few weeks of a cut or trim the ends become scraggly and uneven. Evening up these ends will make the hair look thicker and more attractive.

Frequency of Shampooing

How often should I shampoo? Will frequent shampooing cause hair loss?

You should shampoo as often as necessary to keep your hair looking good and your scalp comfortable. This may range from daily to weekly, depending on how oily your hair is, physical activities, environment, hairstyle, and scalp problems.

Those who have oily hair, exercise daily, or live or work in dirty environments may need to shampoo daily, while others need to shampoo less frequently. Once or twice a week is usually sufficient. When hair begins to look dull, limp, or lusterless, or loses its set, or when the scalp begins to itch, it's time to shampoo.

Frequent shampooing will not cause hair loss. However, daily shampooing of very dry hair and/or overzealous manipulation (excessive brushing, rubbing, etc.) can cause hair breakage that may be mistaken for hair loss.

The Hair-Brushing Myth

Will brushing hair 100 strokes a day make it grow faster and look better?

No. The need to brush hair 100 strokes a day is one of the common hair-care myths. In fact, it may produce the opposite effect by actually damaging hair, thereby causing it to break, develop split ends, and look drab and dull.

That's not to say that brushing hair is undesirable. Brushing helps to keep your hair and scalp clean by loosening and removing dust, grime, hairspray residue, and dead cells. It distributes oil along the hair shaft to add shine and gloss. And it's more gentle than combing for removing snarls and tangles from hair.

Just don't brush excessively or too vigorously. Too vigorous brushing can irritate the scalp. Usually about 20 gentle strokes is all that's needed to keep hair neat and attractive.

The one time you should be very careful about brushing is when the hair is wet. Wet hair is very elastic and may snap when stretched. It should be gently combed with a wide-toothed comb with smooth edges and blunt ends.

Nylon Versus Natural-Bristle Brushes

Does it matter whether I brush with a nylon or natural-bristle brush?

It's not very important what type of brush you use as long as the tips of the bristles are rounded and you don't brush excessively.

Natural-bristle brushes, which most often are made from boar hairs, have naturally tapered, rounded tips. The bristles are soft and flexible. The cut edges of nylon filaments used for nylon brushes may be rough and jagged unless they are polished and rounded off. The filaments may be quite stiff. The stiff, rough, jagged edges can contribute to split ends, hair breakage, and scalp irritation.

Cheap nylon brushes are more apt to have rough edges, since polishing them off would add to the manufacturing costs. You should be able to determine if the edges are rough or too stiff by rubbing the brush across the palm of your hand.

Hair Loss/Alopecia

Normal Hair Loss

I'm sure I'm going bald because my hair is coming out by the roots. I can see the roots on the ends of hairs that fall out.

Don't worry, your hair is not coming out by the roots. You are probably seeing "club" hairs, the hairs that are normally shed during the resting phase of the hair growth cycle.

After a hair grows for a period of time (normally two to six years on the scalp), it enters a transitional period for about three months, stops growing, and separates from the root (papilla). The hair develops a clublike tip on the scalp end and is eventually shed. Then a new hair forms, initiating a new growth cycle. Normally about 15% of the hairs on the head are in the resting phase and may shed.

Since club hairs are no longer firmly attached to the scalp, they are easily dislodged by washing, combing, and brushing. If the hair is still in the follicle when the new growth cycle begins, the new hair will push it out. It's perfectly normal to shed about 50 to 100 hairs per day. Some people mistakenly think that the club-shaped tip of a resting hair is the root and that the hair will not be replaced. When the hair has a clublike tip, you know it's a normal hair that has been lost. Hairs that don't have the normal club tip are being broken by overmanipulation or damage, or have been pulled out. Excessive or abnormal hair loss may be due to many factors, as discussed in the following exchanges.

Causes of Excessive Hair Loss

Please discuss causes of excessive hair loss. I don't know if my hair loss is due to illness, diet, or medications.

Excessive hair loss can be due to a wide variety of causes. Individuals who notice that they are shedding hair after combing or brushing or that their hair is becoming thinner or falling out should consult a dermatologist, who can determine if a specific disease is present and whether the problem will respond to medical treatment. The dermatologist may evaluate a patient's hair problem by asking questions about diet, drugs taken within the last six months, family history of hair loss, any recent illness, and care of hair. The dermatologist may ask a female patient about her menstrual cycles, pregnancies, abortions, and menopause. After examining a patient's scalp and hair, the dermatologist may check a few hairs under a microscope. In a few cases, additional laboratory tests, including drawing some blood for analysis and performing a scalp biopsy, may be necessary.

Between six weeks and three months after a person has any illness accompanied by a high fever, he or she may be shocked to see a lot of hair falling out. This hair loss is usually temporary, with normal growth resuming within a few months.

Abnormal thyroid gland function—both hyperthyroidism (excess secretion by the thyroid gland) and hypothyroidism (a deficiency of thyroid hormone secretion)—can cause hair loss that is usually reversible with proper treatment.

Various drugs may also cause reversible hair shedding in a small percentage of people. Examples of such drugs are some anticoagulants, some anti-gout and anti-arthritis drugs, some antidepressants, some beta blockers (for controlling heart problems and high blood pressure), vitamin A in high doses, and birth control pills.

Hormonal abnormalities in females can result in alopecia, along with other problems such as acne, hirsutism, obesity, and infertility. (Only occasionally are hormonal abnormalities the cause of hair loss in males.) If the hormonal abnormality is corrected, normal hair growth usually resumes.

Major surgery may result in increased hair shedding within two to three months after the operation. The condition reverses itself with a few months. Victims of a severe chronic illness may experience prolonged hair shedding.

Other causes of abnormal hair loss, such as childbirth, are dis-

Since spontaneous regrowth of hair usually occurs, no treatment may be necessary in the less extensive types of alopecia areata. However, it is best to consult your dermatologist to discuss treatment. This may include the application of creams or injections for the hairless areas. Hair transplantation is not an option since the transplanted area can also develop alopecia areata.

Often, in limited cases of alopecia areata, the hair can be restyled to cover the bald areas. Wigs or hairpieces solve the problem for others. When alopecia areata involves the whole scalp (alopecia totalis), a special wig may be required, as there is no hair to which to anchor a normal wig. Special wigs that have suction-cup bases or adhesive attachments to anchor the wig firmly to the scalp are available.

Female-Pattern Alopecia

My mother's hair is very thin now that she is in her 70s. Does this mean that I will also have this problem?

Possibly. Many women develop diffuse thinning of the hair as they grow older. This persistent form of hair loss is referred to as female-pattern alopecia (androgenetic alopecia) and is similar to male-pattern baldness. The pattern of hair loss may resemble that of male baldness with a receding hairline, but most often there is diffuse thinning across the entire top of the scalp, progressing more slowly than in men. It may first become evident after menopause. Women practically never go totally bald. Everyone, men and women, has less hair as they age.

Heredity plays a role in both female- and male-pattern alopecia. The trait is inherited from both mothers and fathers—in men, more from their mothers, in women, from their fathers. The fact that your mother's hair is thinning means that you may also experience thinning as you get older.

The most practical way to conceal female-pattern alopecia is with clever hairstyling. The modern treatments for male-pattern baldness, such as hair transplants, are occasionally recommended.

Hair loss in younger women is usually one of the temporary forms discussed elsewhere in this chapter. Normal regrowth can be expected once the underlying cause is corrected. If diffuse hair loss cannot be associated with one of these causes, medical consultation is advisable. A good endocrine survey, examination, and history are indicated. Treatment with hormones and other internal medications may be necessary.

cussed elsewhere in this chapter. You can write to the American Academy of Dermatology, 1567 Maple Avenue, Evanston, Illinois 60201, for more information on hair loss.

Hair Loss from Cornrows and Pigtails

Can tight plaiting of the hair, as in cornrows or pigtails, cause hair loss?

Yes. Any type of prolonged traction on the hair, especially that produced by cornrows and pigtails, can cause a temporary form of hair loss called traction alopecia. Tight ponytails and sleeping with tight rollers are other causes. Hair loss continues for three to six months, gradually stopping; then the hair slowly begins growing again. If these hairstyling procedures are carried out for many years, however, permanent hair loss may result. In some cases, the hairs may simply be broken off close to the scalp from the traction.

This hair loss is most commonly seen along the front and sides of the scalp where the hair is under the greatest tension, but in the case of cornrows may occur all over the scalp between the cornrows. Some hairs will be pulled out, others broken off. Such loss occurs only after repeated use of these styling methods; it does not occur from occasionally wearing these styles.

Pregnancy and Hair Loss

I have noticed an excessive loss of hair since the birth of my son two months ago. Is this hair loss permanent? Can anything be done about it?

This type of hair loss, known as postpartum alopecia, is common and temporary. While a woman is pregnant she does not lose as much hair as usual. However, after delivery, an abnormally large number of hairs are thrown into the resting phase of the growth cycle and shed.

The increased hair loss becomes evident about two to three months after delivery, when some women may see vast amounts of hair coming out in their brushes and combs. The increased shedding lasts for about one to six months. Normal hair growth usually resumes. Such hair loss may also occur after a miscarriage or an abortion.

Not all new mothers experience postpartum hair loss, and not all women will notice increased hair loss with every pregnancy.

Treat your hair gently and manipulate it as little as possible; brush with a soft, natural-bristle brush, shampoo gently, and pat your hair dry instead of rubbing it. Wear a soft, natural hairstyle that does not require pulling or overmanipulation. Be patient—the hair loss rarely lasts for more than four months.

Hair Loss and the Pill

Can oral contraceptives cause hair loss?

A very small number of women experience temporary hair loss while taking oral contraceptives; more often it occurs after discontinuing them.

Women who lose hair while taking oral contraceptives may be predisposed to hereditary hair thinning and this may be accelerated by the male-hormone-like effects of some of the agents in the pill.

When a woman stops using oral contraceptives, she may notice that her hair begins shedding after two or three months. This shedding may continue for six months, at which time it usually stops. A reversal and restoration of scalp hair occurs six to 12 months after shedding stops.

Hair Loss and Diet

How does diet influence hair loss?

Diets that are severely deficient in protein will influence hair growth, in part because hair is composed primarily of protein. It is essential for people of all ages to eat an adequate amount of protein to maintain normal hair production. Protein is found in meat, chicken, fish, eggs, milk, cheese, soybeans, tofu, grains, and nuts.

Vegetarians, people who go on crash diets that exclude protein, and anorexia nervosa victims who eat tiny amounts of food may develop protein malnutrition. Starvation will produce gross malnutrition. When this occurs, there is a tendency for the diameter of hairs to be reduced and ultimately for the hairs to go into a resting stage. Massive hair loss may then occur two or three months

later. This condition is reversible and preventable by eating adequate amounts of food with a high-protein content.

Certain diets can lead to iron deficiency anemia, which can cause hair loss. However, the belief that hair loss is related to a simple vitamin deficiency has no basis in fact. No single vitamin has been shown to have any pronounced influence on hair growth. Overdosage of vitamins, especially vitamin A, can have toxic effects. If you think you have a nutritional deficiency you should consult a physician. Any great deviation from normal nutrition for any length of time will result in a temporary hair loss.

Alopecia Areata

I suddenly developed two bald spots on my head about the size of a half dollar. The doctor told me I have a condition known as alopecia areata. What is this disorder? Will I go completely bald?

Alopecia areata is a form of baldness affecting about 1% of the population. It usually begins with one or two round bald spots on the scalp that may vary from the size of a dime to a half dollar or larger. The onset is sudden, and the spots may enlarge as surrounding hairs loosen and shed. In most cases only a few spots appear, and hairs stop falling out after a few weeks. However, the disease may progress and the hairless areas merge to result in total baldness. In some cases hair may also be lost on other parts of the body, such as the eyebrows and eyelashes.

In most cases involving limited patchy areas, hair regrows spontaneously after several months. The new hairs may initially lack pigment and have a finer texture than usual, but eventually they become entirely normal. Even in extensive forms of alopecia areata, full spontaneous regrowth may occur. However, the longer the disorder lasts, the less chance there is for regrowth. The more extensive it is and the earlier in life it begins, the more likely it is to persist.

The cause of alopecia areata is unknown. Some experts believe it is an autoimmune disease (self-allergy); i.e., the body reacts to the pigmented hairs as it would to foreign bodies. It is not an infection, nor is it contagious. There is some tendency for alopecia areata to run in families. It has been claimed in some cases to be related to severe emotional stress. However, this has never been proven. In most cases, no cause can be found. It does have a tendency to recur.

Male-Pattern Baldness

Please clarify just exactly what does and does not cause male-pattern baldness. Is it due only to heredity, or do things like dandruff, oiliness, vitamin deficiencies, and poor blood circulation play a role?

Male-pattern baldness (MPB) accounts for over 90% of all cases of permanent hair loss in men. It occurs in 40% of men between the ages of 18 and 39, and 94% of men more than 80 years old. There are three primary factors: heredity, male hormones, and age.

You must have a hereditary predisposition to develop MPB. The genes are inherited from both the father's and the mother's sides of the family. Men have a tendency to inherit this trait more from the mother's side of the family. If your parents, grandparents, aunts, uncles, brothers, or sisters have experienced hair loss with aging, you are a likely candidate for MPB. The extent of baldness and age of onset vary from family to family and from one individual to another within a family. Sometimes the trait will skip generations, sparing some members of a family.

Male hormones (androgens) must be present for male-pattern baldness to occur. Eunuchs do not go bald. Individuals with MPB don't have an excess or a deficiency of androgens; it appears that in those individuals genetically predisposed to MPB, the hair follicles on the scalp are more sensitive to the amount of male hormones produced. What also puzzles researchers is why androgens cause the growth of facial and pubic hair but cause loss of hair on the top of the scalp.

The age at which MPB begins influences the extent of hair loss. Men who begin to lose their hair in their late teens and early 20s are more apt to develop more extensive baldness than those who begin to lose hair in their 50s.

The other factors you mention play no role in MPB. Common baldness is not caused by poor blood circulation in the scalp, so massaging it to increase blood circulation is useless. Likewise, wearing hats or tight headbands will not constrict the blood supply, causing baldness.

Nutritional deficiencies have not been shown to cause ordinary male-pattern baldness. There are no special vitamins, minerals, or other food supplements that will influence MPB.

Excessively oily hair or severe dandruff play no role in MPB. Excessive hair manipulation, shampooing, coloring, and permanents cause hair to become dry and brittle, and to break off close to the scalp, but future hair growth is not affected.

Don't waste your money on the various over-the-counter and salon treatments promoted for the cure of baldness. They are worthless. If you can't stand to be bald, either invest in a well-fitting hairpiece or consult a dermatologist about treatments that are helpful for certain cases of MPB. These include surgical procedures such as hair transplants. These treatments are discussed in the following questions and answers.

Topical Treatments for Baldness

How effective are the various products you can purchase over the counter for application to the hair and scalp for the treatment of baldness?

These products are a waste of money, as noted in the previous answer. None of them will have any effect on male-pattern baldness. If you listen closely to the commercials and carefully read the advertisements, you will note that they do not claim to prevent or cure baldness; the federal government prohibits such claims. What these products promise is to keep your hair in the best condition for as long as you have it. Some of them coat the hairs, making them appear thicker, but they do not affect hair growth. There has been an influx of new products of this type in the last couple of years due to the prescription drug minoxidil. This treatment is discussed in the following question and answer.

Minoxidil for the Treatment of Baldness

How effective is minoxidil for the treatment of baldness?

Minoxidil was originally marketed as a drug to be taken internally for high blood pressure. Because of its numerous, potentially serious side effects when taken internally, it is reserved for cases of high blood pressure that do not respond to other treatments. One side effect noticed by patients taking minoxidil for high blood pressure was the development of excess hair on the body. This led to its use for male-pattern baldness. When applied topically for MPB, side effects appear to be minimal because the concentration is low in the topical drug and the drug is absorbed poorly through the skin. However, patients are carefully monitored for changes in blood pressure and cardiac abnormalities. Changes in heart rate have been reported by Canadian researchers.

Minoxidil was approved by the FDA as a prescription treatment for baldness in 1988. It does not help most cases of male-pattern baldness. It has been shown to grow cosmetically acceptable hair in only 20% of patients. One cannot predict the drug's effectiveness on any individual patient. Minoxidil is most effective for early-stage baldness involving the crown. For many individuals, the hair that regrows is too short and fine to provide any cosmetic benefit. Men who are younger, have been bald a shorter period of time, and have a smaller area of baldness are more likely to respond to minoxidil therapy.

Twice-daily applications of minoxidil, at 12-hour intervals, for at least four months are required before any significant growth appears. Dermatologists recommend treatment for six to 12 months before accepting failure. Once initiated, the therapy must be continued indefinitely to maintain any degree of improvement. When treatment is stopped, hair loss returns.

It is an expensive and rather time-consuming therapy that requires commitment on the part of the patient. The cost of the drug and the physician's care is predicted to be in the range of $80 to $100 per month.

Minoxidil is by no means a wonder drug that solves the problem of male-pattern baldness. It should be emphasized again that the current data indicate that only a small percentage of those who use it will be helped. But it has opened the door for the investigation of other topical drugs, some of which may be even more beneficial for those with male-pattern baldness.

Hair Transplantation

I'm considering hair transplantation for my receding hairline. Please provide details on the procedure and the results that can be expected.

Hair transplantation, a surgical treatment for male-pattern baldness, was developed over 25 years ago by a dermatologist.

In this technique, hair-bearing plugs of scalp from areas not likely to be affected by baldness, such as the sides and back of the head, are transplanted to bald areas of the scalp. The hair at the donor site is clipped and cleaned, and a local anesthetic is injected to numb the area. The recipient site (the bald area) is also cleaned and anesthetized. Using a small, circular, sharp punch, the dermatological surgeon removes small plugs of bald scalp from the recipient area and discards them, leaving circular openings in the scalp. Next, plugs of hair-bearing skin are removed from the donor site and placed in the recipient holes. Each donor plug contains from four to about 15 hairs. Anywhere from 20 to 50 plugs are generally transplanted in one session. Each session lasts about one to one and a half hours.

If necessary, some of the recipient and donor sites are stitched to control bleeding. Then a pressure bandage encircling the head may be put in place for 24 hours. There may be some pain and swelling for about 24 to 48 hours after the procedure.

Following transplantation, care must be taken not to mechanically disturb the transplants. Their secure attachment to the scalp takes about two weeks, so vigorous activity should be avoided during that time.

Dark scabs may form at the site of transplants. These scabs will fall off in two to three weeks. The transplanted hairs in the plugs also fall out as the trauma of surgery causes the hairs to go into the resting phase of the growth cycle. About three months later, new hairs begin to grow, retaining the characteristics of hairs in the donor site.

Donor sites heal within two weeks after transplantation. Because these sites shrink during the healing process, they are covered by overlying and surrounding hair. Therefore, large numbers of grafts can be obtained without creating obvious bare spots. However, new hairs do not grow in these spots. The total number of hairs on the head remains the same; you are simply redistributing the existing hairs to create a more cosmetically acceptable appearance.

Several grafting sessions are usually necessary to provide enough coverage of the bald areas. These may be performed at two- to eight-week intervals. Transplants can be performed on a weekly basis, providing the grafts are put into different areas.

The total number of transplants needed depends on the extent of baldness, the abundance of donor hairs, and the patient's capacity to tolerate the procedure. Pain is usually mild. A minimum of 100 grafts usually is needed to show any cosmetically apparent improvement. The average number of grafts required is 150 to 250 but may go as high as 400 if there is sufficient donor hair. Smaller grafts can be inserted between larger grafts to give a more natural appearance, especially along the hairline.

In the properly selected patient, the cosmetic results can be quite satisfactory. But hair transplantation is not suitable for all cases of baldness, and the degree of success varies. Ideally, hair transplantation should be initiated at a time when hair loss has not progressed very far. Transplants can then be added in small numbers, as needed.

No one should undergo hair transplantation without considerable information on the procedure and the expected results. It requires several months and may cost several thousand dollars. Not everyone is a suitable candidate, even if he can afford the time and money.

If you want to consider hair transplantation, select your dermatological surgeon carefully. Hair transplantation requires expertise and experience.

Scalp Reduction and Flaps

How do the procedures known as scalp reduction and flaps compare with hair transplants?

These procedures may be used along with hair transplants or alone to minimize baldness.

Scalp-reduction surgery may be utilized to reduce the area of baldness on the top of the scalp before transplantation is performed. It is especially useful when the bald area is so large that it cannot be adequately covered by the available donor grafts. Under local anesthesia, a portion of the bald scalp is simply removed surgically to reduce its overall size. Care must be taken not to remove an area so large that adequate closure is impossible. The remaining scalp area is then sutured together. After it has healed and had time to stretch and loosen, scalp reduction can be repeated, if necessary. Hair transplantation can then be performed.

Flap surgery may be utilized instead of hair transplantation to cover a bald area. In this procedure, a pedicle flap (a large thick flap of hair-bearing scalp) is cut free from the scalp except for a pedicle, or stalk, that remains attached. A flap of scalp the same size is removed from the bald area, and the flap of hair-bearing scalp is rotated on its stalk to cover the bald area and then sutured into place. The donor site is sutured and heals with a linear scar that can be concealed by surrounding hair.

Flap surgery carries more risks and requires a skilled physician to achieve satisfactory and aesthetically acceptable results. Therefore, this procedure has not gained the popularity of hair transplants. It is a more formidable procedure, and its failures present bigger problems.

Hairpieces

I'm considering a hairpiece to cover my male-pattern baldness. What information can you provide about them?

A good, well-fitted hairpiece can provide the most practical, economical alternative for many men who don't want to appear bald.

There are different types of hairpieces; they vary in price and quality. They may be made with human hair or synthetic fibers. The appearance of a hairpiece depends on the skill of the person who cuts, trims, thins, tints, and fits the hairpiece. While some of the ready-made pieces can give good results with expert fitting and styling, the best—but most expensive—hairpiece is one custom-made of human hair.

There are several basic types of hairpieces:

1. A "hard top" hairpiece has a hard plastic base into which hairs are inserted. This type of hairpiece usually maintains its shape better and has a longer life. Negative features are that it is heavier and may be uncomfortable in warm, humid climates.
2. A "soft mat" hairpiece has a synthetic fiber mesh base to which hair is tied. The soft mat is usually more comfortable in hot, humid climates, but tends to lose its shape faster and does not last as long as the hard top.
3. A "front lace" hairpiece has a specially treated, transparent, synthetic mesh that extends slightly forward from the main body of the hairpiece. When properly glued to the front of the scalp, it is difficult to see under normal circumstances. This type of hairpiece requires extra time for careful application and generally requires more care than the other types.
4. Partial hairpieces are available in many varieties. They have a small net base to which human or synthetic hair is sewn to give good coverage of limited areas.

Special wigs are available for individuals who are totally bald. These wigs have suction-cup bases or adhesive attachments to anchor the wig firmly to the scalp.

You must also decide on the type of hair to be used in your hairpiece. While human hair is more expensive, it usually looks more natural. It must be tinted periodically as it is subject to fading from sunlight. A hairpiece using synthetic hair fibers is less expensive initially and involves less cost for upkeep. Synthetic hairs are not affected by changes in temperature and humidity. Hairpieces with synthetic fibers are much easier to care for. But they will not look as natural.

Before investing in a hairpiece, shop around and compare prices. Check out the reputation of the seller through friends, former customers, and the local Better Business Bureau. Examine warranties and find out what recourse is available if you are not satisfied with the hairpiece. Most people invest in two hairpieces so they have one to wear while the other is being cleaned.

Hair Weaving

What is hair weaving? How satisfactory is it for baldness?

In this procedure, color- and texture-matched human hair is woven, braided, or knotted into the natural hair. The woven hair is then trimmed and styled to blend with the client's own hair. Since a base of hair is required for the procedure, hair weaving is used to conceal thinning or to alter the natural hairstyle.

In skilled hands, the results of hair weaving can be excellent. However, there are several disadvantages. Since your natural anchoring hairs continue to grow out, the hair weave gradually lifts away from the scalp; it must therefore be redone every four to eight weeks. This incurs repeated cost for as long as the weave is maintained. Shampooing and caring for the scalp and natural hair underneath the hair weave can be difficult. Finally, the tension created by tight braiding of the anchor hair may produce traction alopecia like that resulting from wearing tight pigtails or cornrows. Hair breakage may also occur.

The advantage of hair weaving is that, as a purely cosmetic procedure, it can be removed at any time. You can swim, exercise, and perform other daily activities without fear of the weave coming loose or falling off as can occur with a hairpiece.

Hair weaving is a complex procedure requiring special skill and should therefore not be undertaken lightly. If you want to have your hair woven, find an established, experienced salon so you can be assured of the best results. Also, since you will have to return for refitting of the weave every few weeks, you want to be sure the salon will still be in operation.

Hair Implantation

What is your opinion of hair implantation as a treatment for baldness?

This procedure is not recommended. It is potentially dangerous and generally useless.

One of two procedures may be utilized. In one, synthetic hair fibers are stitched into the scalp. In other other, sutures or other types of anchor points are implanted in the scalp by a physician. Later, a technician attaches a hairpiece or tufts of hair to the stitches or sutures.

Although these procedures seem to provide instant hair, many problems exist. There may be a marked reaction in the scalp, with redness, soreness, and infection. Continuous discomfort is not uncommon. When infection occurs, the sutures or hair implants must be removed; the infection leads to disfiguring scars. The implant may also be sloughed off as a result of the infection.

If no scalp reaction occurs, daily combing and styling of the hairpiece may eventually cause the stitches or sutures to pull out. Another disadvantage of the implantation technique that involves sewing a hairpiece to the scalp is that cleaning beneath the sewed-on hairpiece is very difficult; often an unpleasant odor develops from the accumulation of dirt and oil.

The Food and Drug Administration and state governments have taken action resulting in the closing of most salons offering these services.

3

Other Hair Problems

Facts About Dandruff

What causes dandruff? What's the difference between dandruff and seborrheic dermatitis?

Dandruff is so common that some experts consider it to be normal. Everyone suffers from dandruff to some degree, and the point at which it becomes a source of annoyance is a matter of personal sensitivity. It's only when dandruff becomes noticeable or the scalp becomes too itchy that most of us become concerned.

The outer layer of skin (the epidermis) is constantly replacing itself. Cells are formed at the base of the epidermis and gradually migrate to the surface, where they are shed. This generally takes about a month. An accelerated turnover of the cells on the epidermis of the scalp results in dandruff. As long as the cells are shed individually they are not noticeable, but when cells clump together to form larger flakes they become obvious.

Why cells clump together instead of being shed individually is unknown. If the scalp is excessively dry, what is perceived as dandruff may actually be dry, flaking skin.

Seborrheic dermatitis is sometimes thought of as merely a more severe form of dandruff, but it seems to be a different condition in that there is redness, itching, and inflammation as well as flaking. It may occur in such areas as the eyebrows, the sides of the nose, around the ears, or the chest, as well as on the scalp. Seborrheic dermatitis often requires medical attention for control. Other skin problems such as psoriasis and eczema, which can be confused with dandruff or seborrheic dermatitis, may require totally different treatment.

Frequent shampooing may be adequate to control simple dandruff. More often, it's necessary to use one of the many medicated shampoos promoted for control of dandruff. These products are discussed in the following question and answer.

Dandruff Treatments

There must be hundreds of different brands and kinds of dandruff preparations to choose from. What do you recommend?

You're right; store shelves are filled with a variety of shampoos, conditioners, lotions, tonics, and gels for the treatment of dandruff. Many of them will help, but none will cure it. And no one treatment is best for everyone.

Shampoos are the most popular means of controlling dandruff. Any ordinary shampoo used frequently will control some simple cases for two or three days, but more often medicated shampoos or post-shampoo treatments are needed. Most of these products are formulated to help slow down the formation of scales and/or remove existing scales. They can repress the return of more noticeable dandruff for about a week. Active ingredients include pyrithione zinc, selenium compounds, salicylic acid, sulfur, and coal tar. To be effective, the shampoo should be left on the scalp for three to five minutes before being rinsed off.

If dandruff persists or is severe, you should consult a dermatologist. You may have a scalp disorder such as psoriasis, eczema, or seborrheic dermatitis rather than simple dandruff. The dermatologist may prescribe a shampoo or a cream or lotion containing specific medication to control your particular case.

Cradle Cap

What causes "cradle cap" in babies? How should it be treated?

Cradle cap is thought to be a severe form of infant dandruff, but the exact cause is unknown. It may form when a mother neglects to clean an infant's head during bathing for fear of injuring the "soft spot." Grease and scales pile up on the scalp, forming a coating that resembles a cap, hence the name.

Cradle cap is not serious and usually disappears within a few months. It may cause temporary hair loss when hairs are pulled out with the scales. If untreated, it may spread to other areas. Frequent, gentle shampooing usually alleviates the problem. If not, consult a dermatologist.

The presence of cradle cap may indicate that a child will develop seborrheic dermatitis or psoriasis later in life. In fact, cradle cap may be a manifestation of a number of scaling conditions in which the scales adhere to the scalp. Frequently these cannot be distinguished from one another in the infant.

Fine Hair

I hate my fine, thin hair. Isn't there any way I can make it change to thick hair?

Sorry, but there's no way to make normal, fine hair permanently thicker. This is an inherited characteristic, just like color and curliness or straightness. Only in rare instances is fine, sparse hair due to some internal disturbance. For example, such hair in infants or young children may be associated with an inherited metabolic disorder; in adults it may be a sign of malnutrition or starvation.

Cosmetic treatments offer the best solution for fine hair. A body permanent designed especially for fine hair adds body and helps hair sets last longer. Some people find that bleaching or tinting adds body and texture, but care must be taken not to overprocess and damage hair. Certain mousses and styling gels also help to add body. Short hairstyles are generally preferable to long, straight styles.

Green Hair

Help! My blond hair has turned green. How can I get rid of it?

Green hair is an uncommon but distressing problem that most often affects naturally blond, dyed-blond, and white hair. On rare occasions it affects brunettes.

Green hair is most often caused by increased concentrations of copper in tap water and swimming pools. Corrosion of copper

27

pipes causes the problem in tap water, while copper-containing algicides are responsible in pools.

Much less common causes of green hair are industrial exposure to cobalt, chromium, and nickel; topical treatment of scalp ringworm with yellow mercuric oxide; and the use of a tar shampoo.

Conditions that make the hair vulnerable to copper absorption include physical damage (from, for example, frequent use of hot blow dryers, curling irons or curlers, overbrushing, and sun exposure) and chemical damage (from bleaching, frequent permanent waving, straightening, and alkaline shampoos).

There are no simple home remedies to remove green hair. But a professional beautician may be able to remove the green color with a shampoo containing chelating agents such as edetic acid. Try to avoid further exposure to copper-containing water, and don't damage your hair further with chemical or physical abuse. (See the section on minimizing swimming-pool damage to hair later in this chapter.)

Can Gray Hair Regain Color?

Is it possible for gray hair to regain its natural color?

Normal graying of the hair, as occurs in most individuals with aging, is permanent. The process cannot be reversed. The only time color can return to gray hair is when graying results from disease. The hair may permanently or temporarily regain its original color when the patient recovers, but only in new hair growth. The hair that has already formed will remain gray. Thus, some hairs may be gray at the tips and pigmented closer to the scalp. Or hairs may have alternating bands of gray and color as the pigment-forming capacity of the hair root changes with the severity of the illness.

Disorders that may cause graying, and in which color may return, include: endocrine gland disorders, injury or disease of the nervous system, physical or mental shock, vitiligo, alopecia areata, and some severe illnesses such as malaria and influenza.

Turning Gray Overnight

My grandfather swears that a friend turned gray overnight during the war. Is this possible?

Although folklore, stories such as your grandfather's, and even medical articles describe hair turning gray overnight, it's really impossible. There has never been a fully documented, completely convincing scientific report to support this claim. More logical explanations for apparent instant graying are illustrated with the famous case of Marie Antoinette, who is supposed to have turned gray the night before she was beheaded by the guillotine. It is more likely that her gray hair either grew out during her imprisonment when she did not have access to hair dyes (dyes did not last long back then) or had been concealed with a wig (large, elaborate wigs were always worn in public during that period).

Hair color is provided by special pigment-forming cells at the root, which deposit color pigments in hair as it is being formed. Once formed, hair becomes a dead, hardened shaft of protein. The only way that hair could turn gray overnight would be if a substance penetrated the hair shaft from root to tip and removed all the pigment. No such substance is known. Cosmetic hair-bleaching products bleach hair only above the scalp.

Individuals who have a mixture of gray and pigmented hairs may seem to go gray overnight if they suddenly shed all their pigmented hairs, leaving only the gray hairs. This can occur in an unusual form of hair loss known as alopecia areata. Alopecia areata has a tendency to selectively affect pigmented hairs, sparing gray hairs (see Chapter 3 for more details about alopecia areata). Of course, the hair will also be sparser in such cases.

In ordinary graying, the pigment-forming cells become inactive and future growth is unpigmented (gray). But the hair that is already formed remains pigmented. Generally, graying is a gradual process as hair follicles scattered over the scalp become inactive a few at a time. Thus, a person first develops streaks of a "salt and pepper" scattering of gray and does not become totally gray for several months or years. Some people never turn totally gray.

Oily Hair

My hair is so oily that I must shampoo every day or two. I worry that such frequent shampooing is harmful. Isn't there any way to permanently get rid of the oiliness?

No. The most practical way to control excessively oily hair is to shampoo more frequently, daily if necessary. This is not harmful.

Use a shampoo formulated especially for oily hair that has good oil-removing qualities. Commercial shampoos vary widely in their cleansing, oil-removing qualities. Some have high detergent or drying characteristics while others are designed to be less efficient cleansers. You may prefer a shampoo that does not include oily conditioning ingredients. Shampoo twice if necessary, leaving the second lather on the hair for about five minutes before rinsing thoroughly.

If you need a post-shampoo conditioner, select one that is oil-free or has less oily properties. A short haircut will make frequent shampooing easier and there will be less hair to accumulate oil.

There is no safe, simple way to permanently reduce the oiliness. Hyperactivity of oil glands connected to hair follicles within the skin are responsible. There are no external treatments that will slow down the activity of the glands to reduce the oiliness. All these products can do is remove the oil that has reached the surface.

Infrequently, excessive oiliness may be associated with endocrinological problems such as polycystic ovaries or adrenal hyperactivity resulting in the increased production of androgens (male hormones). The diagnosis and treatment of such problems require expert medical evaluation.

How to Minimize Damage from Daily Swimming

I swim almost every day at the health club. The chlorine in the water is wreaking havoc on my hair. What do you suggest?

Daily exposure to chlorine and water has a drying effect on the hair that can lead to various problems: hair breakage, excess tangling, and a dull, lusterless appearance. The problem is compounded by the necessity of shampooing daily to remove the chlorine. The following hair-care program can be helpful.

1. Shampoo with a mild shampoo formulated for dry, damaged hair. Don't lather up twice. Be sure to thoroughly rinse out all residue.
2. Apply a conditioner after every shampoo. It will deposit a light film on the hair to counteract dryness, add gloss, and make it easier to comb.
3. Wrap your hair in a towel and gently pat dry. Wet hair is very fragile and easily damaged by vigorous rubbing.

4. Gently comb the hair with a wide, blunt-toothed comb. Never brush wet hair. Work out tangles by combing gently, working from the tips toward the scalp.
5. Wear a short, simple hairstyle that requires minimum manipulation. If you must color, permanent wave, or chemically straighten your hair, have it done by a professional hairdresser to minimize further damage.

The Cure for Split Ends

I saw an ad for a hair product that claims to cure split ends. Will it work?

No. The only way to get rid of split ends is to cut off the hair beyond the point of the splits. Split ends occur when the individual cell layers of the hair shaft separate. There is no known way to permanently stick them back together. A hair product such as a conditioner may temporarily "glue" split ends together, but the ends will separate again after a few hours or days, especially after the next shampoo.

Long hair is more apt than short hair to be plagued with split ends because it has been subjected to more abuse over a longer period of time, so one way to minimize split ends is to wear a short hairstyle. Regular haircuts should keep split ends under control.

See the question and answer on basic hair care (Chapter 1) for more details about how to avoid/minimize split ends.

Singeing the Hair

I read about a famous hairdresser who singes the ends of hair after cutting to avoid split ends and make hair healthier. Is this desirable?

Absolutely not. In fact, singeing can damage hair and promote split ends. Singeing burns the tips of hairs so they are more susceptible to splitting.

The notion that singeing is good for the hair is based on the erroneous belief of the past that the hair has a hollow canal through which flows a nourishing, life-giving fluid. Thus, cutting would open the end of this canal, releasing the nourishing fluid and causing the hair to die. Singeing is supposed to seal the tip so the life-giving fluid does not escape.

This theory is totally false. The hair shaft does not have a hollow canal that contains nourishing fluids. We now know that the shaft is actually a dead structure that cannot be nourished. Split ends occur when the hair is abused (by excessive heat, for instance) and the individual cell layers of the hair shaft separate. Once split ends have developed, the only way to get rid of them is to cut the hairs off beyond the split.

It is surprising in this day and age, with the scientific knowledge that exists about hair, that anyone, especially a professional hairdresser, would still practice such a useless, damaging procedure.

Help for Dull, Drab Hair

What can I do to bring shine and bounce back to my dull, lusterless hair?

Many factors may contribute to dull, drab hair so the first step is to determine the cause. Dull, drab, lusterless hair may be caused by damage to the cuticle layer from excessive dryness or oiliness, damage from the environment (sun, chlorine in swimming pools), overzealous use of heat-styling applicances (blow dryers, curling irons), excessive or improper use of bleaching, waving, straightening, or hair-color products. Sometimes hair becomes dull, limp, and droopy from buildup of such hair-care products as mousses, gels, hairsprays, shampoos, and conditioners. Dull hair can also be associated with illness, internal disorders, or dietary deficiencies.

If the hair is damaged, you will have to allow new, undamaged hair to grow out to permanently bring back shine and gloss. In the meantime you can obtain more manageability and luster by shampooing with a gentle shampoo formulated for damaged hair and by using a post-shampoo conditioner. Lusterizing gels and mousses or sprays are now available that temporarily restore the glossiness to hair. Coating the hair with an oily or oil-like material will add luster and sheen much as oiling or waxing wooden furniture does.

If your hair suffers from the "greasies" brought on from buildup of hair products on the hair, shampooing the hair for a week or two with a gentle, straightforward, nonconditioning shampoo should remove the buildup and bring back bounce and gloss.

If you suspect your problem is due to a dietary deficiency or an internal disorder, consult a dermatologist.

4

Hair-Coloring Products

Types of Hair-Coloring Products

I'm not happy with my hair color and I would like to change it, but there are so many different types of hair-coloring products on the drugstore shelves that I'm confused. Can you enlighten me on the subject?

You are not alone in wanting to change your hair color. It's estimated that about 50% of all women color their hair, and an increasing number of men do too. Anyone would be confused by the variety of products, from many different manufacturers, that fill the hair-coloring section of the average drugstore.

Today's consumers are not dependent on professional care exclusively to color their hair. Hair-dye manufacturers in recent years have increased the ease, simplicity, and convenience of application. Many kinds of color change can be achieved successfully with home-use products; others, especially drastic color changes, are still best left to the professional hairdresser.

If you understand how the different types of hair-coloring products work you can begin to sort out the packages on the shelf. There are basically six types: 1) temporary colors, 2) semi-permanent colors, 3) permanent oxidation dyes, 4) lead acetate dyes, 5) vegetable dyes, and 6) bleaches. Bleaching may be done as a preliminary step to semi-permanent or oxidation dyeing or alone. There are also specialized bleaching techniques such as frosting and streaking.

You will find a detailed discussion of each type of coloring process in the rest of this chapter. With an understanding of the pros and cons of each type of product you can then decide just what kind of color change you want. If you decide to color at home with one of the products from the drugstore shelf, it is absolutely essential to read and follow directions exactly.

Temporary Colors

I would like to add a little color to my hair to brighten it, but I'm afraid to go right to a permanent dye in case I don't like the effect. What can I expect from a temporary coloring product?

A temporary coloring product may be all you need. These products primarily add highlights and brightness to natural color, tone down gray or yellow hair, and blend streaked hair. They cannot produce drastic changes in hair color. They offer a good way to test a color since they are easily removed with a single shampoo.

There are two types of temporary colors: rinses and high-intensity color products. The rinses color the hair only lightly, while high-intensity color products impart deeper shades to the hair.

Rinses are available primarily in liquid form. After it has been applied, the hair is styled, without rinsing. When used in high concentrations the effects are not natural. At least one brand of spray-on temporary color in this category is available.

Dyes used in rinses are usually certified colors, that is, purified synthetic dyes that have been tested for safety and certified by the Food and Drug Administration for use in food, drugs, and cosmetics. These dyes are quite safe, so no patch test requirement appears on the product label. Rinses also contain a mild acid that enhances the uptake of dye by the hair.

Some products may contain other synthetic dyes in addition to certified colors so the label includes a precautionary statement and instructions to perform a preliminary patch test. (Patch testing is discussed in more detail later in this chapter.)

Most of these products are designed to provide styling and conditioning effects in addition to color.

Some products are available as sprays, mousses, or gels. Some, promoted as "fun" colors for the hair, are available in bright red, blue, gold, silver, pink, and other exotic shades.

All the temporary products deposit the dye or colored particles on the surface of the hair, rather like a coat of paint. There is little or no penetration of the dye into the hair structure. For this reason the high-intensity temporary colors may rub off on pillows and clothes. Perspiration may cause some "bleeding" of color onto the skin. While temporary colors are somewhat resistant to water, they are completely removed with a single shampoo.

Semi-Permanent Coloring Preparations

What are the pros and cons of semi-permanent dyes? How safe are they?

Semi-permanent colors have several advantages. They last longer than temporary colors but are removed after four or five shampoos, so you aren't stuck with the color if you don't like it. The products are easy to use, look quite natural, and are less apt to cause allergic reactions than permanent oxidation dyes. The disadvantages are that the results are not permanent and they cannot be used to achieve a shade lighter than the original color of the hair.

These products contain organic dyes that are mostly specially designed dyes with penetrability and fastness for hair. They do not require an oxidizing agent (hydrogen peroxide) or ammonia as do oxidation dyes, so they do not require mixing prior to use. This means they are simpler to use, and milder than oxidation dyes. They are applied directly to the hair and thoroughly worked in like a shampoo. Most are liquids but a few are available in mousse form. Because the color penetrates into each hair, it is completely colored and there is no rub-off as with temporary colors. Depending on the length and frequency of application, they can be used to gradually color the hair or to give immediate effects.

Semi-permanent dyes are available in a complete range of colors from ash blond to natural black. However, they cannot make hair lighter. A variety of gray shades, such as smoke, steel, or platinum, are also available. In fact, these products are most often promoted to cover gray hair (when less than 40% of the hair is gray and evenly distributed) or to enhance the gray and remove the yellow tones. They may also be used to refresh the color of the hair between applications of permanent oxidation colors, or to add highlights to natural hair. They usually are not recommended for use on bleached hair.

The incidence of allergic reactions to semi-permanent dyes is very low and they often are used by people who are sensitive to the oxidation dyes. Nonetheless, a precautionary label appears on each package that directs the consumer to perform a patch test before each use. If you decide to use one of the preparations, be sure to follow these directions and apply the patch test before every application. (See detailed discussion of patch testing elsewhere in this chapter.)

Permanent Oxidation Dyes

How do permanent oxidation dyes work? Can I use one at home or must I go to the beauty salon?

Permanent oxidation dyes are the most popular hair-coloring products for both home and professional use. They are the only such products that are truly long-lasting. They come in a complete range of natural colors, from the palest blond to jet black. They also are the only products that can lighten as well as darken hair. These products are sometimes referred to as tints.

The term "oxidation" is applied to these dyes because the final color in the hair is produced by an oxidation reaction. The product must be mixed with a developer or oxidizing agent immediately before use, and the oxidative, chemical reactions take place in the hair. The dye mixture is thus trapped within each hair, providing more or less permanent effects.

These products are sometimes called "para dyes" or "amino dyes" because they contain paraphenylenediamine, or closely related materials, as the coloring substances to be oxidized. The formulation may also contain ingredients designed to make the colorants penetrate readily into the hair shaft, to give the preparation structure and stability, and to provide lubricating and conditioning properties.

The developer is usually 6% hydrogen peroxide in water or in a creme formulation. Occasionally other oxidizing agents, such as urea peroxide, are used in the form of tablets or crystals to be dissolved in water. Since hydrogen peroxide is also a bleaching agent, it can remove some of the natural color from the hair at the same time the new color is being produced. That's why permanent oxidation dyes can lighten hair color. However, if an individual desires to go more than two or three shades lighter, the hair must first be pre-bleached to remove more or all of the natural color. The package directions usually provide a clear explanation of how much lightening can be expected. The directions will indicate that if your hair color is color X it can go no lighter than color *Y*. The package directions will also state that a preliminary color test should be performed on a lock of hair. It is important to carry out this test since unexpected color reactions may result when hair is damaged or has been previously colored with some other types of dyes.

Professional products are usually creme formulations applied by the technique known as "parting and sectioning." In contrast, for home use, "shampoo-in" products are more popular because they are easier to use. As soon as the developer is mixed with the dye formulation, the product is shampooed into the hair all at once. This innovation has increased the home use of these dyes. However, shampoo-in products do not generally cover gray as completely as creme formulations. When complete gray coverage is desired, the parting and sectioning technique with a creme formulation is preferred.

All kits of oxidation dyes for home use also contain a final rinse aimed at both thoroughly removing all traces of the oxidation product and conditioning the hair. Most products available today not only produce color of good quality but also perform well in imparting such conditioning effects as enhanced gloss and feel.

Since the results of oxidation dyeing are more or less permanent, new hair growth must be periodically dyed to match the dyed hair. Hair grows about ⅓ to ½ inch per month, so "retouching" is required about every six to eight weeks or the contrast between new growth and dyed hair will become noticeable, especially if the hair has been lightened. Care must be taken to avoid overly exposing the hair that is already dyed to the new dye application or there will be an unnatural buildup of color in this portion of the hair. With creme formulations it is possible to dye only the new hair growth. In this "retouch" method, the hair must be parted and sectioned carefully and the formulation then applied to each section. This is difficult to do oneself, so retouching is best done by a professional. If a shampoo-in product is used for retouching, greater care must be exercised to prevent a gradual buildup of color toward the ends.

Finally, and perhaps most importantly, a preliminary patch test must be done before every application of an oxidation dye. These products have a greater potential than other dyes to cause allergic sensitization, that is, development of an allergy that will cause a skin reaction (dermatitis) to develop when the dyes come in contact with the scalp of a sensitized individual. These reactions may be minor or quite severe. *Therefore, you must perform a patch test before each and every application of an oxidation dye,* especially since an allergic reaction may not develop until the dye has been used for months or years. This subject is covered in more detail later in this chapter.

Lead Acetate Dyes

What do you think about lead acetate dyes?

Lead acetate dyes are among the oldest hair coloring preparations, having been used since ancient times. But their appeal today is limited; they are used mostly by men seeking to conceal gray hair. These products are sometimes called progressive dyes or "color restorers" because they produce a gradual buildup of color with daily application.

The metallic salts in lead acetate dyes react chemically on the hair to produce color pigments that are deposited on the surface of the hair as a coating.

The chief advantage of these dyes is their ease of application; often they are simply combed in each day until the desired depth of color is reached. The color is then maintained by application every few days.

There are many disadvantages to the lead acetate dyes. Because the coloring is deposited on the outside of the hair like a plating, the natural luster is obscured. Another disadvantage is that these dyes tend to produce dark and intense color rather than muted, lighter shades that are more becoming. Once applied, the dyes are difficult to remove, and they are totally incompatible with other coloring products, especially oxidation dyes. In addition, lead acetat dyes may interfere with permanent waving.

The dyes apparently are quite safe and do not cause allergic reactions. Over the years, fears have been expressed about the toxic absorption of lead from such products, but such concerns seem to be unfounded. However, these products should not be used to dye beards or moustaches close to the mouth. This presents a potential danger of ingestion of lead, which may cause internal problems.

Vegetable Dyes

Is henna the only plant dye? How do these dyes compare to other types of dye?

Vegetable dyes are probably the oldest type of dye in existence, having been in use for thousands of years. This long period of use has established their safety as well as their cosmetic limitations.

Actually, although these hair dyes have traditionally been referred to as vegetable dyes, other plants have served as the source for the dyes down through the centuries. Indigo, camomile, and extracts from wood (redwood, logwood) and nuts (gallnuts, walnuts) have all been used to dye the hair, but only the henna plant is used today.

Henna is generally applied as a "pack"—the ground leaves and stems of the plant are made into a paste with hot water, and the paste is applied directly to the hair for various lengths of time. However, the color produced is a harsh, unnatural orange-red that becomes even less pleasing as the color is intensified with repeated applications. Henna also has an adverse effect on texture, making the hair stiff and brittle. There have been attempts to soften the shade by adding metallic salts, and even a synthetic self-oxidizing dye precursor (pyrogallol) that gives a drabbing effect. Such products are called "compound hennas." A truly natural henna plant dye is usually identified as "pure henna" on the label.

There was a resurgence of interest in henna on the part of some "high fashion" hairdressers in the early 1980s, but the popularity seems to have faded as the unnatural effects and shortcomings became obvious with multiple applications. More natural-looking red shades can be obtained with semi-permanent or permanent oxidation dyes.

The interest in henna relies on its natural origins and the fact that it is very safe. It has no apparent toxic characteristics and almost never causes allergic sensitization.

Why Patch Test?

Why is it important to do a patch test before using some dyes? How is the patch test performed? How do you know which dyes require patch testing?

Many hair-coloring preparations may cause allergic sensitization. An individual may develop an allergic sensitivity to these products *at any time* so that subsequent exposure will produce a skin reaction (dermatitis) on skin areas that come in contact with the dye. Repeated applications may increase the sensitivity.The rash may be no more than a red itching rash or it may be severe, causing itching, discomfort, swelling about the eyes, and redness and crusting of the face, neck, and scalp. In rare instances, a generalized reaction over the body may occur.

Federal law requires that labeling for all oxidation dyes, semipermanent colors, and some temporary colors bear the following warning:

> Caution: This product contains ingredients which may cause skin irritation on certain individuals and a preliminary patch test according to accompanying directions should first be made. This product must not be used for dyeing the eyelashes or eyebrows; to do so may cause blindness.

Instructions for the patch test are given with each package. In general, about 24 hours—preferably 48 hours—before the hair dye is to be used, one applies a drop of the dye formulation (or if it is an oxidation tint, a mixture of the dye and developer in the proper proportions) on the inside forearm near the elbow. If any reddening or swelling develops over the next 24 to 48 hours, the dye should not be used.

The patch test should be performed before each use of the dye since one may be insensitive to the dye initially but develop sensitivity during subsequent applications. Professional hairdressers sometimes perform the patch test only before the first application, not repeating it for subsequent colorings. Such a practice is not to be condoned.

Sensitivity to one color or brand of dye may indicate a sensitivity to all preparations of the same type, for example, oxidation dyes. Therefore, anyone who develops a positive patch test from one oxidation dye should not use any other brand or shade of oxidation dyes. In such instances, one may be able to use another type of dye, such as a semi-permanent one, but a patch test still must be done to rule out sensitivity to the other type of dye.

Even a negative patch test does not absolutely exclude the remote possibility that an allergic reaction may occur at the time of hair dye application. One small loophole exists: A person can become allergic to a dye and yet show no reaction at that application. The next exposure (patch test or actual use) will be followed by a reaction. It is even possible, although remotely, that one may be sensitized by the patch test procedure itself.

It is worth mentioning that the physical symptoms of an allergic reaction are only temporary.

Toners

What are toners?

Toners are specially formulated "light" dyes that are applied to the hair after bleaching to provide a more desirable shade and to neutralize the red tones that are often left after bleaching. The entire process of bleaching and toning is sometimes called a "double process."

The dyes may be of the oxidation type, like the permanent tints, or they may be nonoxidation toners, similar to semi-permanent dyes. In either case, a patch test is required to ensure that the individual is not sensitive to the dye.

Hair Dyes for Men

Are there any differences between hair dyes promoted for men and those for women?

Hair dyes promoted to men may be formulated with shades and scents that are more acceptable to men, but the basic formulas are identical. Men generally prefer drabber shades than women. Traditionally, men have been the primary users of metallic dyes, but today many are switching to the semi-permanent coloring products because the shades look more natural and hair texture is better. These dyes are discussed elsewhere in this chapter.

Frequency of Hair Dyeing

How often is it safe to dye the hair?

You must be referring to permanent oxidation dyes and/or bleaching since other products do not last very long. These procedures should not be carried out more frequently than every three or, preferably, four weeks. Since hair grows only about $\frac{1}{3}$ to $\frac{1}{2}$ inch per month, this frequency should be adequate to keep new growth color concealed. Excessive use of permanent oxidation tints, and especially bleaches, may cause the hair to become damaged and fragile, leading to breakage and loss of texture.

Don't try to change your hair color too frequently or too drastically, especially at home. If you want to go from dark brunette to ash blond have the coloring done by a professional.

Bleaching to Lighten Hair

I want to lighten my hair several shades. Will I have to bleach it? How much damage will this cause to my hair?

If you want to lighten your hair by more than two or three shades, you must first bleach it to remove some or all of the color. This is referred to as pre-bleaching as it is generally followed by application of a toner. Toners are special tints in blond shades that tone down the bleached hair, giving it a more desirable shade (toners are discussed elsewhere in this chapter.)

Pre-bleaching should be done with a commercial hair-bleaching product, which usually consists of three components. Six percent hydrogen peroxide in liquid or creme form is added to a hair-lightening lotion that contains a mild soap and ammonia, a necessary ingredient to produce bleaching. For faster and higher bleaching action an accelerator (booster, activator) is often added. Accelerators are forms of persulfate salt in varying degrees of solubility and alkalinity.

Any bleaching damages hair, making it more porous and brittle. This is not necessarily discouraging, provided one can maintain the hair at a reasonable, attractive, and soft-textured level. Regular conditioning is recommended to protect the hair from weathering and handling. The degree of damage increases with the degree of lightening, as discussed next.

Dark Brown to Pale Blond

My hairdresser says that I may have to bleach my hair twice to go from dark brown to pale blond. Will this damage my hair?

Some damage is almost inevitable when hair color is drastically lightened. To go from dark brown to light blond your hair must be pre-bleached to remove most of the color. (This procedure is sometimes called "stripping".) It is advisable to do it in several steps, both to avoid too great a stress on the hair and to allow the user to make sure he or she wants to reach a very pale blond.

This is a very drastic treatment for the hair. It may become very porous, weak, brittle, and strawlike. In order to keep the hair in the best possible condition, it is strongly recommended that the bleaching be done by a proficient expert, using high-quality products.

If bleaching is continued for a long time, the hair may become extremely dry and brittle, with a tendency to break off close to the scalp. Such hair is very fragile and must be handled very gently. Tips on caring for bleached hair follow.

Tips to Minimize Damage from Bleaching

I really must have blond hair, and that means bleaching it. How can I minimize damage?

All bleaching results in some damage to the hair. To minimize this damage follow these tips:

1. Bleaching should not be done too frequently. Do not bleach hair more than once a month.
2. Minimize physical punishment of the hair from brushing, combing, curling, teasing, and other mechanical handling.
3. Keep bleached hair conditioned. Always apply a conditioner after shampooing to minimize tangling and aid wet combing. Conditioners also add luster, softness, and manageability.
4. If you use a blow dryer, set the heat level no higher than medium. Try to avoid hot curling irons or use them infrequently. Heat damages hair.
5. Don't use permanent wave products on highly bleached hair. This is adding another chemical assault and potentially increasing the damage to the hair shaft. This is especially true when the hair has undergone multiple bleaching to achieve a very light shade. If you must permanent wave your bleached hair, have it done professionally. Using a mild permanent-waving preparation developed specifically for bleached hair will minimize additional damage.

Gentle Hair-Lightening Products

What do you think of "gentle lighteners"?

The so-called "gentle lightener" has become popular in recent years. These products do not produce the degree of lightening that traditional bleaching products do, but they are less damaging and cause little discomfort to the scalp.

Frosting, Tipping, Painting, and Streaking Hair

What's the difference between frosting, tipping, painting, and streaking? Are there any advantages over regular bleaching?

These are all double-process techniques that involve bleaching selected strands or streaks rather than all of the hair. Each technique gives different effects. Frosting gives an overall salt-and-pepper effect by bleaching selected strands all over the head to blend with the darker hair. Tipping is a variation of frosting in which only the tips of selected strands are bleached. If only one or two wide sections or strips of hair are bleached, the process is known as streaking. In hair painting, bleach is applied to the outside of the hair with a paintbrush in either chosen or random patterns. These techniques can produce interesting or dramatic effects, especially on dark hair.

Two methods are available for frosting and tipping. In one, a special plastic cap with tiny holes is placed on the head and fine strands of hair are pulled through the holes and then bleached. In the other method, a few strands of hair are selected and placed on a square of aluminum foil, bleach is applied starting about ¼ to ½ inch from the scalp (or just to the tips), and the foil is wrapped around the hair until the bleaching process is completed. The degree of frosting or tipping is controlled by the number of strands bleached. The foil technique is slower, but some people prefer the effect achieved. It is the only technique used for streaking.

The bleach used for all these techniques is very active and comes in the form of a paste for accurate positioning. After bleaching, a toner can be applied to provide a more desirable shade.

There are several advantages to frosting, tipping, or painting compared with overall bleaching. Since the bleaching solution does not come into contact with the scalp there is no danger of irritation. In fact, frosting and tipping can offer an alternative to those individuals who want blond hair but whose scalp is irritated by regular bleaching. All of the hair is not involved so only those hairs that have been bleached are damaged. The procedures do not have to be repeated as frequently as for all-over bleaching, so damage to the bleached hair is minimized.

Reactions to Persulfate Boosters in Hair Bleaches

Do persulfate boosters in hair bleaches pose any health hazards?

Yes, ammonium persulfate can present hazards for a very few susceptible individuals. Reactions can range from mild to severe, from immediate to delayed.

There may be an immediate tingling and burning sensation on the scalp and face as the product is applied to the hair. The scalp and face may become red and swollen and hives may appear in the local area. The hives sometimes become generalized. An individual may also develop a red, itchy, and crusty rash called a contact dermatitis. Other possible reactions are dizziness, faintness, loss of consciousness, and even shock. Some people suffer asthma attacks or rhinitis (runny noses) from exposure to persulfates. Severe reactions require immediate medical attention, and possibly hospitalization. These reactions have been seen only following the use of ammonium persulfate.

Ammonium, sodium, and potassium persulfates are commonly used to speed up or "boost" the action of hair bleaches. They are referred to as "boosters," "accelerators," "proteinators," "strengtheners," or "fortifiers." They have a strong oxidizing action that accelerates the bleaching action and enables hair to be bleached to extremely light shades. Persulfates also make the hair more porous or receptive to the dyes or toners that are commonly applied after bleaching to achieve the final desired color.

The persulfate booster is always added separately to the peroxide solution in an extra step just before use. For home use, the persulfate boosters are often sold in separate packets with instructions to add one or more packets to the peroxide bleach solution. Professional hairdressers often purchase the persulfate in bulk packages.

Anyone who experiences a persulfate reaction should seek medical attention. The physician can prescribe various medications to bring the reaction under control. *If there is a reaction, persulfates must be avoided in the future.* The hair can still be bleached, but without the persulfate booster the process will take longer and it may not be possible to obtain extremely light shades.

Advice to Beauticians About Persulfate Boosters

What advice can you provide to me, a professional beautician, about persulfate boosters?

The persulfate booster is always packaged separately, as a "booster," "accelerator," or similar term. It is added to the bleach solution just before use, its purpose being to boost the action of the bleach. While these products are safe for the majority of clients, you should be alert for reactions in susceptible individuals (including yourself).

If a client develops swelling and redness of the face and scalp and hives immediately after hair bleaching, the reaction is almost always due to the persulfate booster.

Should a client complain of itching, dizziness, or faintness during a hair-bleaching procedure, stop and obtain immediate medical attention.

Once a client reacts to the booster, such a reaction is likely to recur every time the individual is exposed. Such individuals may still be able to bleach their hair with a peroxide bleach without persulfate; however, the bleaching will take longer and an extremely light shade may not be obtainable.

If you develop any of the symptoms discussed in the previous question and answer when you are exposed to persulfate boosters you too must avoid them in the future. Published reports on persulfate reactions describe beauticians who have suffered reactions ranging from hand dermatitis to urticaria (redness, swelling, hives) and asthma attacks.

5

Hair Waving/
Straightening

Permanent-Waving Procedures

Please explain how permanent waves work. What's the difference between regular perms and "acid" perms?

Permanent waving today is performed almost exclusively with what are called "cold wave" products. These products, introduced in the 1940s, revolutionized permanent waving and made home permanent waving possible for the first time. Older permanent waving techniques required the use of a special heat machine.

Permanent waving is a two-step process that changes the configuration of some chemical bonds (called sulfide bonds) in the hair. In the first step, these chemical bonds are broken so that the hair, which has been wound on curlers, will accept the new curled shape. In the second step, the bonds are reformed in the curled shape by application of a neutralizing solution that "hardens" the hair in the new curled configuration to produce "permanent" waving.

The hair is shampooed, then wound on curlers. The diameter of the curlers, their position on the head, and the number used determine the tightness of the curl and the final style. When all the curlers are in place, each curl is saturated with waving lotion.

Since the waving lotion can irritate the skin, care must be taken to avoid contact with the surrounding skin.

The waving solution is usually left on the hair for about 10 to 20 minutes, with the exact time determined by the condition of the hair, the strength of the waving solution, the environmental temperature, and the degree of curling desired (one curl is usually tested for curliness). After the rolled hair has been rinsed thoroughly with water, a neutralizing (oxidation) lotion is applied, saturating the hair on each roller. After a few minutes the hair is rinsed with water and the curlers removed.

There are basically four types of cold waving preparations available today:

1. Traditional cold waves with alkaline ammonium thioglycolate
2. Traditional cold waves with a lower pH
3. Acid permanent waves
4. Light permanent waves

The traditional cold wave utilizes an alkaline waving solution containing ammonium thioglycolate (pH of 9–10) and a neutralizer containing sodium bromate or hydrogen peroxide.

A variation of the traditional cold wave utilizes a thioglycolate-based waving solution with a lower pH (7.5–8.5). The prepared hair is covered with a plastic cap to entrap body heat, which accelerates the reaction. These two types of cold wave perms are available for both home and professional use. All ammonium thioglycolate perms have an unpleasant odor.

Acid permanent waves, introduced in the early '70s, are not really cold waves. Glyceryl monothioglycolate is used at a pH of 7–8. After the solution has been applied to the curled hair, the scalp is wrapped in a plastic cap and the subject is placed under a hair dryer. The reaction is then neutralized as in the traditional cold wave technique. More recently, acid perms have been introduced that do not require the heat of a hair dryer for processing. The scalp is simply wrapped in a plastic cap during processing, utilizing entrapped body heat. These new acid perms are considered milder than the hot acid perms. Both types of acid permanent waving must be performed in a salon; these products are not available for home use.

The fourth type of cold waving preparation is called a "light wave" because it is much less active. The active ingredient in these products, which are sold only for home use, is a weak reducing agent with a pH of 6–8. The scalp is covered with a plastic cap during processing to retain body heat. The neutralization process is the same as for other cold wave permanents. Light waves have the advantage of not being malodorous but they are less popular; only a few brands are available.

The safety of the various permanent waving techniques is discussed in the following answer.

Reactions to Permanent Waving

Does permanent waving damage hair? What about allergic reactions? I heard that acid perms cause more reactions than other types.

Reactions to permanent waving solutions are relatively rare, considering their extensive use.

The most common complaints after permanent waving are brittleness, frizziness, split ends, and breakage of hair close to the scalp. A frizzy or wirelike texture results when too much hair is curled too tightly or too many narrow-gauge curlers are used. Excessive hair breakage occurs from too much chemical action on the hair. This can occur from using too strong a solution or leaving the waving solution on too long (overprocessing).

A poor wave, or "take," may occur if the waving solution is too weak or is not left in contact with hair long enough. A scant wave with poor body will result when the hair is too short to permit at least one full turn on the curler or when the hair is not wound tightly enough around the curler to produce adequate stress.

Hair damage can be minimized by having the permanent done by an experienced beautician. Precautions are discussed in the next question and answer.

Allergic reactions to traditional cold wave permanent waves containing ammonium thioglycolate are *extremely* rare. If an allergic reaction does occur, it may be due to other hair products such as shampoos or conditioners used at the time of permanent waving. Skin irritation is more common when the waving solution is allowed to run onto the skin surrounding the scalp. These reactions range from redness (erythema) to more serious inflammation of the skin.

Irritant and allergic reactions on the hands of hairdressers and on the face, neck, scalp, and hairline of their customers from the "acid" permanent wave have occurred; however, the incidence is still considered low.

The bisulfite "light waves" also occasionally produce allergic reactions.

(See the previous discussion for details about the different types of permanents.)

Professional Versus Home Permanent Waving

Are the results of home permanents and professional permanents comparable?

That depends on the type of curl and styling you desire and how closely you follow directions for home use. The condition of the hair is also important.

Permanent-waving solutions intended for home use are usually weaker than those used in beauty salons, a precaution taken by the manufacturer to reduce the possibility of hair damage in the event that the consumer does not follow the directions—the cause of most problems with home permanents. The consumer may not have properly rolled the hair on the curlers or applied the right amount of waving solution to each curl. If the waving solution is left on for too long, overprocessing results; if not long enough, the hair will not be curly enough. If the neutralizer is not correctly applied, the hair will not be properly neutralized. This may result in brittleness, frizziness, split ends, and breakage close to the scalp, or failure of the curls to be permanently waved.

For these reasons, it is best to solicit the help of a friend for home permanent waving. The friend can help roll the hair on the curlers, apply the waving solution and neutralizer, and time the procedure.

If you plan to use a home preparation, be sure to carefully read and follow the directions for use. And don't assume that different brands can be used in the same manner. In fact, the directions for one brand may change from one use to the next.

Finally, be sure your hair is in good condition before you begin. Damaged or overbleached hair demands special attention if good results are to be achieved without further damage. If your hair is damaged, you may prefer to have it waved professionally. A good beautician will be able to evaluate the condition of your hair and determine if it can withstand the permanent-waving process. The professional beautician also has a wider range of products to choose from and the expertise to determine which process is best for your hair and the style you desire.

Waving Bleached Hair

Can I safely have my bleached hair permed?

Bleaching is a chemical process that results in a permanent modification of the hair fiber. The tensile strength of the fiber is reduced and the hair becomes more porous. The amount of change depends on the original hair color and the amount of lightening. Very dark hair that is highly bleached will be more fragile than light hair bleached to the same shade.

Permanent waving adds further chemical modification to the hair. Whether the bleached hair can withstand the added changes produced by permanent waving depends on its condition. While special permanent-waving solutions are available for bleached hair, damage may still be unavoidable. If there is any question about the fragility of hair resulting from the bleaching, the permanent-waving solution should be tested on one lock of hair before it is applied to the whole scalp.

If you want to permanent wave bleached hair, it is best to have the procedure done by a professional.

Permanent Waving and Pregnancy

Is it true that permanent waving is not successful during pregnancy?

There is no scientific basis for this opinion, even though some beauticians state that permanent waves are less successful at this time.

Since the hair that is visible above the scalp is dead, it is not affected by changes in the body such as pregnancy. The hair can be altered only by such external treatments as permanent waving, straightening, dyeing, or bleaching.

Sometimes the degree of oiliness of the hair changes during pregnancy (it may increase or decrease) because the activity of the scalp's oil glands may be altered. This cound possibly affect the texture or feeling of the hair and its appearance, but changes in the degree of oiliness should not affect the action of permanent waving preparations, if the hair is properly shampooed first.

Care of Permanent-Waved Hair

Does permanent-waved hair require any special care?

Permanent-waved hair has undergone structural alteration. Among the changes produced is disruption of the highly reflective outer layer (the cuticle) of the hair. The degree of disruption is proportional to the harshness of the chemical treatment. The hair feels rough, has less shine, and is difficult to groom in comparison to untreated hair. The cuticle cells of individual hairs are elevated, causing the hairs to snag and tangle easily. The hair has less body, and the electrostatic charge is increased, which makes the hair difficult to manage. In the wet state, the more porous hair absorbs greater quantities of water so that it is temporarily heavier and clumsy to manage.

Such hair may benefit from the use of a slightly acidic shampoo. These shampoos cause less swelling of the hair shaft when it is wet than do alkaline shampoos and may make the hair less porous by temporarily flattening the raised cuticle scales. Using a conditioning rinse after shampooing is another aid for damaged hair. Conditioners add body to the hair, modify the surface of the hair to make combing easier, and decrease the buildup of electrostatic charge that causes flyaway hair. Conditioners add softness and shine to the hair that has been damaged by waving. (See Chapter 6 for more information on shampoos and conditioners.)

Permanent-Wave Failure

What can cause a permanent to fail to "take"? My hairdresser claims it's not her fault.

Permanent waves fail for numerous reasons. Hair texture is one important factor. Fine, limp hair usually resists permanent waving, as does hair that is wiry, brittle, or damaged.

Some permanent-wave lotions must remain on the hair for a long time to alter the chemical bonds and wave the hair; if the wave solution is removed from the hair too soon, insufficient waving results. If the neutralizer is not applied or not left on long enough, or does not work for some reason, the chemical bonds will revert to their previous noncurled form. Neutralizers that contain hydrogen peroxide will sometime become weaker or inactivated before use; the neutralizer will then be ineffective and the wave will not take. Thorough rinsing is important before applying a neutralizer to eliminate any residual reducer.

Most products are made in large, individual batches, and a manufacturer would receive many complaints about failure if there were something wrong with a batch. (In the absence of such complaints, the problem probably occurs in the beauty salon.) You may want to contact the manufacturer about the failure of your permanent. You can get the name and address from your hairdresser.

Electric Rollers

What are the pros and cons of electric rollers? Any advantages to mist rollers over plain electric rollers?

Electric rollers have become a popular means of curling hair. Many people do not bother with the traditional wet, set, dry styling procedure. Instead they blow dry their hair and then use electric rollers or curling irons to provide some curl.

Electric rollers are usually hard plastic rods of two or three different sizes, in sets of 20 to 24. Rollers are available with blunt-toothed or smooth, flocked surfaces. The latter are gentler to the hair because the hair is less apt to become tangled on the curler during removal. In most models the rollers are electrically heated on upright metal mandrels in a plastic container. Electric curling units have automatic cut-off switches designed to turn off the heating element when the rollers have reached a certain temperature. Most have a thermal safety fuse as well. This prevents the rollers from becoming so hot that the hair would be burned and damaged.

Some electric roller sets have the capability of acting as mist (steam) rollers when a small amount of water is added to a small container in the plastic case. As the rollers are heated, the water vaporizes and permeates the rollers as a steam mist. Mist rollers add a small amount of moisture to the hair, which in turn aids in producing the temporary set. Curling "sticks" are the latest innovation in electric rollers. These are long, flexible plastic rods that are wound around the hair to provide more body and waves rather than actual curls.

None of the electric rollers will provide as tight or long-lasting a set as the regular wash, set, dry procedure, but they seem to be satisfactory for many modern hairstyles.

Electric Curling Irons

Curling irons are very fast and convenient, but I wonder about possible damage to the hair. What precautions should one exercise when using a curling iron?

Electric curling irons are very popular today for adding curl and lift after blow drying because many popular hairstyles do not require the traditional wash, set, dry procedure. Busy lifestyles that call for more frequent shampooing and leave no time for weekly visits to the beauty salon for traditional sets have also added to their popularity.

The heat emanating from the curling iron breaks some of the weaker hydrogen bonds of the hair, making it possible to temporarily curl it. Most curling irons have a medium and a high setting. The lower setting is less apt to burn the hair or scalp but will not produce a tight curl.

Some curling irons have caps on the end of the curling stick to which water can be added to turn the curling iron into a mist (steam) curler. The moisture produced aids in forming the temporary set.

Curling irons are much hotter than electric curlers, and scalp damage can result from careless use. Generally, though, there is no need to worry about damage to the hair from modern appliances as most are equipped with a thermostatic control that prevents the appliance from reaching a temperature at which hair damage could occur (about 100°C). Curling irons should not be used daily on hair that has been chemically treated (bleached, permed, straightened).

Curling irons are available with smooth or plastic "brush" surfaces. The problem with the latter is that the hair is more apt to tangle in the bristles, producing damage. Many curling irons come with two or more curling sticks: two sizes for small and large curls, and both a smooth and a bristle surface.

Wave-Setting Preparations

There are so many different wave-setting preparations available—gels, mousses, aerosol and pump sprays, and creams. How do they differ? How can I tell which one is best for my hair?

There has been a revolution in wave-setting products in recent years, led by the clear setting gels and the mousses. But liquid and spray products are still popular with many people.

Most of the modern products are intended to add body and help shape the hair rather than help maintain pre-formed curls. Most are used in conjunction with blow drying and electric curlers or curling irons.

All these products contain various synthetic polymers that help the hair hold styling longer. The ingredients will vary by form (e.g., gel, mousse, or cream), but any of these products should provide satisfactory sets when used according to the manufacturer's directions. The amount of product applied to the hair will determine to a large extent the softness or firmness of the set. Too much product will make the hair dull and result in flaking that may resemble dandruff.

Mousses are really intended to provide body and are most often used in conjunction with blow drying. Gels tend to give harder, stiffer body and are used more often for styles that require stiffness. Most manufacturers provide different formulations for hard-to-set and normal hair. Some incorporate extra ingredients to condition hair, provide anti-static action, or add sheen or luster.

The only way you can determine which type you will prefer is to try various products. The method of application or form of the product may be a deciding factor. Gels tend to be messier to apply than mousses.

If you prefer the traditional wet, set, dry procedure, you may prefer one of the more traditional wave-setting products in liquid or gel form.

Hair-Straightening Techniques

What methods are available for straightening curly hair? How safe and effective are they?

Three methods are used to straighten naturally curly hair: 1) application of pomades or resinous fixatives, 2) passing a heated comb through the hair (hot pressing), and 3) the use of chemical straighteners.

None of these methods is totally safe or effective, especially for extremely curly or kinky hair. All have certain drawbacks. Pomades are simple to use and relatively safe, but they are rather messy and provide only temporary effects. Hot pressing also produces temporary results and is potentially damaging to both hair and scalp. It should be performed in a beauty salon by a professional. Chemical straightening produces longer-lasting results, but some chemical straighteners can cause significant scalp and hair damage. Chemical straightening products are available for both home and professional use. A discussion of each method follows.

Pomades for Straightening Hair

How safe and effective are pomades for straightening hair?

Pomades (heavy oils or petrolatum-type products) plaster the hair against the scalp and remove some of the curliness by strictly mechanical means; there are no chemical changes in the hair. The straightening results are temporary.

Pomades make the hair greasy and are most effective on short hair. They are more popular with men than women.

Pomades occasionally produce a contact dermatitis in people who may be sensitive to the perfume or other ingredients in the products. They may also cause outbreaks of skin blemishes along the hairline, referred to as "pomade acne."

"Hot Pressing" for Straightening Hair

What are the pros and cons of hot pressing? What does this technique involve?

Hot pressing or combing to straighten hair has been widely used, primarily in beauty salons, to temporarily straighten hair.

After shampooing and towel drying, a small amount of pressing oil is distributed throughout the hair. The oil serves as a heat-transfer medium and as a lubricant for hot combing. A metal pressing comb, heated to 300–500°F, is passed quickly through a tress of hair. The high temperature breaks some of the chemical bonds within the hair and permits the hair to be straightened under the tension of hot combing. The hair temperature drops rapidly as the comb passes through, and the broken bonds unite in a new position, causing the hair to retain its new straightened position. The results are only temporary because exposure of hot-combed hair to water, high humidity, or even scalp perspiration causes the hair to revert to its original curly configuration. Thus, hot pressing must be repeated at frequent intervals to keep the hair straightened.

Hot pressing can cause both hair and scalp damage. The hot comb may produce first- to third-degree burns of the scalp or surrounding skin. Faulty technique, carelessness, and too-frequent use of the hot comb can cause substantial hair damage. Hair may break off close to the scalp, resulting in temporary bald patches. (The hair will regrow satisfactorily if further damage to the hair is avoided and the scalp is not scarred, destroying hair follicles.)

Chemical Hair Straighteners

How do chemical hair straighteners work? Are there different types?

Chemical hair straighteners are the only products that will produce long-lasting straightening of visible hair. The principle used is just the reverse of that of permanent waving, in that the hair is straightened rather than curled after the chemical bonds have been disrupted. However, stronger chemicals are usually required for straightening than for waving.

The alkaline straighteners contain the strongly caustic chemical sodium hydroxide. The sodium hydroxide causes the hair to swell and induces breakage and alteration of the chemical bonds in the hair fibers. This action is very rapid, and the fibers relax quickly under the tension of combing. The hair is then rinsed with water to stop the chemical action. Because of the rapid chemical action of these products, they must be left on the hair for no longer than 5 to 10 minutes; otherwise the hair may be seriously damaged. (It is important to exactly follow the directions on the package.) The scalp and skin may suffer first- to third-degree chemical burns from contact with the sodium hydroxide, so the scalp and surrounding skin should be covered with a protective cream.

If alkali straighteners come in direct contact with the eyes, they can cause blindness. Fortunately, these products are usually provided in very thick cream forms, and accidental contamination of the eyes is rare. For safety reasons, alkali straighteners are best applied by professionals.

Follow-up care is elaborate and includes successive applications of moisturizers, curl activators, and oil sheen that saturate the hair and scalp. A plastic cap is worn to bed each night.

Thioglycolate straighteners are a newer innovation in chemical straighteners. They contain the same active ingredient as cold wave permanents, but in higher concentrations. These products are most often used in beauty salons, although a few products are available for home use.

Thioglycolate lotions or creams are applied to clean, damp hair and take from 10 to 20 minutes to break the chemical bonds in hair so it can be straightened. The hair is combed while the straightener is acting in order to pull the curl out. This must be done cautiously to avoid hair breakage. The hair is then rinsed with water and neutralized with an oxidative solution, which rebuilds new bonds to produce hair that is straight instead of curly.

Thioglycolates are irritating chemicals and may cause contact dermatitis of the scalp and surrounding skin. They produce fewer reactions than alkali straighteners, but unfortunately they are not as effective either. The thioglycolates do not break and realign all the chemical bonds of the hair, so that hair does not become as straight.

Hair that has been damaged by prior chemical treatments such as bleaching should not be subjected to straightening. Also, some manufacturers advise against using hair colors that require peroxide on chemically straightened hair.

Bisulfite straighteners are the most recent development in chemical hair straightening. They are most popular for home use, but some professional products are also available. The term "curl relaxer" is used to describe bisulfite products because they do not produce the degree of straightening provided by alkali or thioglycolate straighteners. They are better suited for relaxing curly hair in Caucasians than in blacks.

The bisulfite curl relaxers act in the same way as thioglycolate straighteners. The chemical bonds of the hair are broken and then set in the new, straightened position. After the bisulfite lotion is applied to clean damp hair, the hair is covered with a plastic turban for about 15 minutes. Next, the hair is combed for 15 to 20 minutes to produce the degree of curl relaxation desired. The hair's chemical bonds are then relinked in their new orientation by rinsing the hair with water and then with an alkaline stabilizer (neutralizer) solution. A conditioner is applied to the hair as the final step.

Bisulfite curl relaxers are much milder. They are not as likely to cause a reaction on the scalp and are less damaging to the hair than other types of hair-straightening products. However, manufacturer's directions and precautions must still be carefully followed.

While chemical straighteners straighten the visible hair, it's necessary to straighten the new hair growth every few months. Care must be taken not to double-process hair that has already been straightened, or severe damage and hair breakage may occur. This is difficult to avoid because of the combing technique that is an integral part of straightening.

Precautions/Limitations for Chemical Hair Straighteners

It appears that chemical hair straighteners present some problems. What special precautions should be observed? What can be done for hair damage by chemical straightening?

All the chemical hair straighteners present some hazards and none is completely safe or always effective. With present technology, there is no satisfactory, nondamaging method for changing extremely curly or kinky hair to completely straight hair. Some degree of straightening can be achieved, but some damage will also occur to the hair.

Expertise and caution are bywords for chemical hair straightening. The procedure is more complex and potentially more hazardous than permanent waving because it requires stronger chemicals, increased concentrations of the products, or longer application times. Straightening with alkali or thioglycolate products is best done by a professional, but be sure that the professional is experienced in chemical straightening.

The alkali straighteners will effectively straighten kinky curly hair but may significantly damage the hair and scalp. The thioglycolate straighteners cause less hair damage than the alkali straighteners but are less effective in straightening hair. They may produce scalp irritation.

The bisulfite curl relaxers are less likely to damage the skin or hair than the other types of chemical hair-straightening products. However, these products are not very effective for very curly hair; they are best for straightening Caucasian hair.

If hair has been bleached, color treated, or previously straightened, any straightening must be done with extreme caution.

Whether hair is being straightened at home or professionally, a strand of hair should be tested first according to the manufacturer's directions. The consumer should carefully read and exactly follow the manufacturer's directions and precautions when using a home preparation.

Damage is more apt to occur on long hair that has been subjected to repeated straightening. If hair that has been straightened is damaged, future straightening should be avoided until new, undamaged hair has grown out. If the procedure is repeated, it should be done with extreme caution.

Damaged hair must be treated gently. Limit combing and brushing to the minimum required to keep hair groomed. After shampooing, pat the hair dry; don't rub it. Apply a post-shampoo conditioner to help minimize tangling and restore luster, feel, and manageability. Use a wide-toothed comb to gently comb wet hair; don't brush it. And avoid overexposing hair to the summer sun, since it will increase the hair's dryness and weathering. Periodic oil treatments before shampooing may be helpful. With time, new, undamaged, normal hair will replace the damaged, broken hair.

6

Other Hair Products

The Best Shampoo

Is there really any best shampoo? Is price a good guideline?

Not really. There are hundreds of brands of shampoo to choose from, and new ones hit the market every week. Most of them will do a satisfactory job of cleansing the hair.

The price you pay for a shampoo is a matter of personal preference. But it's not necessary to spend a lot of money to obtain a good shampoo. With expensive brands you are sometimes paying for the "name" and for the advertising/promotional costs of the manufacturer rather than special shampoo qualities. On the other hand, you may need twice as much of some cheap shampoos to adequately shampoo the hair, so in the end the cost could be comparable to that of more expensive, concentrated products.

All shampoos contain a combination of surfactants, which are responsible for the cleansing action. They loosen dirt, oil, and other residues on the hair so they will be rinsed away with the suds. Soap is rarely used as the surfactant in shampoos today because soap interacts with hard water to leave an insoluble soap scum on hair. It has been replaced with synthetic detergents. (Manufacturers avoid using the term "detergent" to describe the surfactants in shampoos because they fear that consumers will mistakenly associate the term with harsh household detergents. In fact, detergency is the process of cleaning.)

There are dozens of different surfactants, with different properties. Some are better at removing dirt while others are best for removing oily deposits. Some don't foam very well; others produce a rich lather. Some leave hair looking better than others. For this reason, shampoo manufacturers generally use two or more surfactants, with one surfactant providing the primary cleansing action while others modify the formula. For example, if the principal surfactant is excellent for cleansing but produces little lather, the manufacturer may add another surfactant to provide added lathering action since consumers associate cleansing with lots of suds. (Actually this is erroneous; you don't need a lot of lather for cleansing.)

Most formulations for oily, dry, and normal hair contain different combinations of surfactants. A shampoo for oily hair should have a surfactant with greater oil-removing qualities than a shampoo for dry hair. But in actual use, consumers often have difficulty judging any differences between such shampoos.

If your hair needs conditioning, use a post-shampoo conditioner rather than a conditioning shampoo. It is difficult for a shampoo to have two diametrically opposed functions—to cleanse the hair and at the same time leave behind a film of pure conditioner. The residue that remains after using a conditioning shampoo will, of necessity, also include some detergent residue. This residue can build up to produce the "greasies," as discussed elsewhere in this chapter.

And don't assume that just because a shampoo is described as "thick" and "rich" that it is better. Manufacturers add thickening or thinning agents to achieve the viscosity or "richness" they want for marketing and aesthetic purposes.

In fact, most of the the ingredients you find listed on shampoo labels are included to provide the aesthetic qualities that often determine which shampoo we purchase. Emulsifiers are added to keep the various ingredients mixed together. Antioxidants can be added to help prevent breakdown when the product is exposed to air. Preservatives are necessary to avoid contamination. Foam boosters are added if the surfactant doesn't provide enough foaming action. Other ingredients may be added to make the product opaque or pearlescent. Finally, color and fragrance are usually included.

The pH of shampoos is adjusted to range from mildly alkaline to slightly acidic. The only time you have to be concerned about the pH of a shampoo is when your hair is damaged. A shampoo that has a neutral or slightly acidic pH causes less swelling of the hair and less roughening of the outer cuticle layer, and this is desirable for damaged hair.

So, in the final analysis, there is no best shampoo. Since hair differs and shampoos differ, the best advice is to try different shampoos until you find one you like. Try inexpensive ones and popular brands. Take advantage of the small trial sizes that most manufacturers sell for a nominal price. When you find a shampoo you like, stick with it—unless your hair changes, presenting different needs.

What About Those Special Additives in Shampoos?

Are there really any special benefits from herbs and other botanicals, eggs, honey, jojoba, aloe vera, henna, and other additives in shampoos?

The shampoo market is very competitive because customers are rather fickle about shampoos, always changing brands. So manufacturers keep adding "special" ingredients to get our attention through advertising. A few years ago it was protein, then balsam and herbs, now various botanicals such as aloe vera and henna are popular. It's claimed that many of these natural ingredients provide special conditioning or rejuvenating qualities, but there is little or no scientific evidence to support such claims. You can't feed or nourish hair: It's dead. Most shampoos have some conditioning qualities, but the primary purpose is to cleanse the hair. Conditioning is best provided by a separate conditioner. Many of the special ingredients are simply part of the fragrance.

More details about shampoos are provided in the previous discussion on shampoos.

Soap as a Shampoo

Why can't I simply use my bar soap for shampooing?

You can, if you have soft water. Unfortunately, most areas of the United States have hard water. The minerals in hard water interact with the fats in soap to produce an insoluble soap scum or residue that makes hair look dull and droopy.

Before the second World War, everyone had to use soap to

shampoo (synthetic detergents were developed during World War II). That's why our grandmothers collected rain water for shampooing and used lemon, vinegar, or beer rinses. These are mildly acidic and rinse away the soap scum.

Today, 99% of all shampoos are based on synthetic detergents because they have very little interaction with hard water and thus leave little or no residue. Acid rinses are unnecessary when these shampoos are used.

Dry Shampoos

Is there any way to cleanse the hair besides using regular wet shampoos? My grandmother has had a stroke and it is difficult to give her regular shampoos very often.

Waterless, or dry, shampoos offer an alternative means of cleansing the hair although they are not as effective as regular shampoos. They are especially useful when illness precludes regular shampooing.

Dry shampoos generally consist of an absorbent powder and mild alkali. They are available as dry powders, aerosol foams (mousses), or waterless liquids. The method of application varies, but in essence, the product is applied to the hair and left for a few minutes. The powder absorbs surface oils, dirt, and odors. Then the product is brushed, combed, or toweled off.

One problem with dry shampoos is availability. They are not very popular so distribution is limited.

Which Conditioner to Use

I'm confused by all the different kinds of conditioners. Are those that contain botanicals better than others? Should I use one that is "self-adjusting"?

Modern conditioners are useful hair-care aids but there are so many different brands, with so many different claims, that it's no wonder you and many other consumers are confused.

The bottom line is that any conditioner will "condition" your hair. They all make hair soft and more manageable, help detangle hair, counteract static electricity that makes hair flyaway, and add shine, bounce, and body to dry, damaged hair. But some perform some of these functions better than others. The following information should help you sort through the various packaging and advertising claims to find a product that meets your particular needs.

First, you must realize that the hair above the scalp is dead, so you can't "feed" or "nourish" it or permanently repair damage. Conditioners can only provide temporary benefits that are removed with the next shampoo. The only way to get rid of damaged hair is to cut it off.

Shampooing removes the natural oily film that acts as a natural conditioner on hair, and may roughen the outer cuticle so that hair tangles more easily and looks dull. If hair is old and/or damaged from physical or chemical abuse, the cuticular surface may be permanently roughened and some of the cuticle may be absent, exposing the inner cortex layer, which may then split into individual fibers (split ends).

Conditioners, when applied after shampooing, deposit on the hair strands an invisible film that smooths the roughened cuticle and may even fill in spots where the cuticle has been worn off. This makes the hair less apt to tangle and easier to comb, and adds shine, body, and bounce.

Most conditioners are "instant" conditioners that are left on the hair for only a minute or so before being rinsed off. They are quite satisfactory for most people, but severely damaged hair may benefit from periodic use of a "deep conditioner" that is left on the hair for 15 minutes or more before being rinsed off.

There are also conditioners for normal, oily, and dry hair, and, recently, conditioners for "mature" hair have been introduced. Theoretically a conditioner for oily hair should have less oil or be "oil-free," but this is not always the case. In one consumer survey, users couldn't distinguish much difference between these different types of conditioners. Conditioners for "mature" hair are simply conditioners that manufacturers have targeted at today's increasing number of older consumers. They don't actually differ from other conditioners as far as conditioning effects are concerned.

Conditioners with various plant extracts such as aloe vera, jojoba, or herbs, or with botanicals such as camomile, or with various flowers, don't provide any special benefits. They act like other oils or proteins. Proteins are helpful ingredients because they stick to the hair, helping to fill in a damaged cuticular surface, not because hair is made of protein.

The fact is that all conditioners are "self-adjusting." The hair absorbs or holds onto conditioner only where it needs it; the rest is rinsed away.

All conditioners add some body to hair because the conditioner coats the hair, thus making it a little thicker. In actual use, it's sometimes hard to distinguish any difference between regular and "extra body" conditioners.

You want to evaluate a conditioner's effect on both wet and dry hair. When hair is wet you want it to comb easily without tangles. When the hair is dry you want it to feel soft, to comb easily, and to not be flyaway. It should have shine and bounce.

Sometimes the final decision in selecting a particular conditioner is made on the fragrance, look, or feel of a product rather than on any real conditioning benefits. Price is also a consideration. Just because a product costs more, it's not necessarily better.

When shopping for a new conditioner, look for the small trial sizes that most manufacturers sell. This will enable you to try the product and be sure you like it before investing in a full size. Or write to the manufacturer for a free sample; most are happy to send you one.

Hopefully, this information plus the discussions that follow will help you steer through the "hype" when selecting a conditioner.

Conditioner Ingredients

The ingredient listings on conditioners are endless. What do all of these things do? Which ones are important?

The important ingredients in conditioners are those that provide the various conditioning actions: detangling, softness, manageability, shine, bounce, easy combing, and flyaway control. The following breakdown may help you distinguish these ingredients from those that are included to provide physical characteristics such as thickness and color, or to support advertising claims. (Specific ingredients listed are simply examples of commonly used ones.)

Ingredients in conditioners and other cosmetic products are listed in descending order of concentration. Water is always the first ingredient listed as it serves as the base for all other ingredients. Is also adds some moisture to hair. The next ingredient listed will have the next highest concentration and thus may indicate the primary conditioning action of a particular product.

Most conditioners contain one or more natural or synthetic oils to lubricate hair strands, reduce tangling, and prevent moisture loss. Mineral oil and lanolin are examples of commonly used natural oils. Jojoba oil, mink oil, and other exotic oils are often touted as providing "special" benefits; however, the benefits they provide are no different from those of other natural oils. Some conditioners, especially formulations for oily hair, contain synthetic polymers such as silicone, dimethicone, and cyclomethicone or acrylics and epoxy derivatives to perform the functions provided by natural oils in other conditioners.

Humectants such as propylene glycol, panthenol, and glycerine help make hair feel soft and bouncy by attracting moisture from the air. Proteins are included in many conditioners, especially those for damaged hair, as these ingredients stick well to hair, smoothing and filling in roughened, uneven surfaces, and temporarily gluing split ends together. The proteins range from hydrolyzed animal protein to such exotics as sea kelp or other "food" ingredients.

Quaternary ammonium compounds, or "quats" as they are commonly called, are important ingredients because they enable the conditioner to form a bond to hair. They also help counteract static electricity and flyaway hair. Stearalkonium chloride and cetrimonium chloride are examples of quats commonly used in conditioners. Ingredients such as citric acid (lemon juice) control the pH of the product.

The rest of the ingredients in conditioners have nothing to do with conditioning. They determine the final look, feel, and smell of the product. There are emulsifiers to keep the oil and water mixed together (glyceryl stearate, polysorbate), thickeners (cetyl alcohol), opacifiers (distearates), ingredients to control consistency (isopropanol), and antioxidants to prevent the product from breaking down when exposed to air [butylated hydroxytoluene (BHT)], preservatives to prevent bacterial contamination (parabens, sorbic acid, methylchloroisothiasolinone), and, of course, color and fragrance.

When to Condition

Do I need to condition my hair after every shampoo?

Not unless you need it. While some people need to condition their hair after every shampoo to keep it shiny and manageable, others need to condition only once in a while. Besides providing gloss and manageability, conditioner helps to protect hair from environmental or handling damage.

If you have normal, undamaged hair worn in a short style you may need to use a conditioner only when your hair is subjected to abuse or adverse weather conditions that can be drying. Some people need conditioners only during the winter months when the humidity is low and hair tends to develop static electricity that makes it flyaway.

You should avoid overconditioning, as this can cause the "greasies," a buildup of residue from conditioners and other hair products, as discussed in the following question and answer.

The "Greasies"

What causes the "greasies"? It seems that after I use a shampoo for a while my hair begins to look dull, limp, and greasy instead of light and fluffy.

The "greasies" is commonly applied to hair that has developed a buildup of residue from overuse of conditioning shampoos, conditioners, mousses, gels, or any of the other products we apply to our hair today.

Consumers have demanded conditioning shampoos because they think they are better for the hair; these shampoos are designed to leave some residue. Then many people use a post-shampoo conditioner, a mousse, or a gel and spray. This residue gradually builds up on the hair, making it dull and limp.

The best way to avoid the greasies is to use a good, simple shampoo that is not loaded with conditioning ingredients. It should remove the buildup of various hair-care products as well as clean the hair. Then apply a separate conditioner if you need one.

Blow Drying

I use a blow dryer practically every day because it's faster to dry and style my hair by this method. But I worry about damage to my hair. Can you provide any tips to minimize damage?

Blow dryers have become the primary means by which people dry their hair today. Blow drying is faster than the traditional wash, set, dry procedure, and some popular hair styles demand blow drying. Done properly, it doesn't have to be damaging to the hair, even when it's done on a daily basis.

Set the dryer on the medium or cool setting and a slower speed. This minimizes the potential for burning or overdrying the hair and scalp and actually makes styling easier. Keep the dryer about

6 to 12 inches from the hair and keep the flow of air moving over the hair. Don't keep the flow on one spot of hair for more than a few seconds or you may burn your scalp. Be careful not to overdry your hair; all hair needs moisture to be pliable. Your hair should still be slightly damp even after it's been styled and dried.

Be especially careful to use lower settings when blow drying permed, bleached, or damaged hair, as it is more fragile. And try to avoid daily blow drying of such hair. Regular use of conditioners can help to minimize further damage.

Hair Sunscreens

Is it beneficial to use a hair sunscreen? Can sun damage hair just as it damages skin?

The hair can become dry, brittle, and discolored from overexposure to the sun. The tensile strength is reduced. Hair that has already been weakened by bleaching or permanent waving is especially vulnerable. The sun also has an adverse effect on the color of dyed or bleached hair.

A good hair sunscreen could help to minimize this damage. Unfortunately, many of the hair products promoted for this purpose may not be very helpful. Many do not deposit enough sunscreen on the hair to provide any screening effects. For example, most of the sunscreen in a shampoo or conditioner is probably rinsed out. Other products, such as mousses or gels, may not contain enough sunscreen to provide adequate protection. Perhaps in the future, manufacturers of hair sunscreens will have to develop measurement terms to indicate their degree of protection, just as sunscreens for the skin must be labeled with their degree of protection via an SPF (Sun Protective Factor) number. (See Chapter 21 for detailed information on SPF and sunscreens.)

Mousses for Hair Styling

What can I expect a mousse to do for my hair? Does it perform the same function as a conditioner?

Mousses are not conditioners; although they provide some conditioning qualities, their primary function is to aid in styling. You may need to use both a conditioner and a mousse, depending on how you want to style your hair.

A new category of hair-styling products emerged when the first mousse was introduced in the early 1980s. While aerosol foam products had been around for some time, many of them felt sticky and did not spread easily through the hair. Mousses are not sticky. They spread evenly through hair, yet they provide good control. They enable you to shape and mold the hair so that it looks natural while it still holds its shape well after drying. However, to hold the hair in exaggerated styles you need a gel, as discussed in the following answer.

Mousses may contain cationic polymers, anionic polymers, or a combination of both. The cationic polymers facilitate styling and combing and make the hair shiny. The anionic polymers fix the hair, giving it more body and fullness.

Although the directions for styling with mousses indicate that they can be applied to either damp or dry hair, they are primarily used on damp hair.

Gel for Styling

I want to style my hair so it will stand up in the front. Should I use a mousse or a gel?

You should use a gel if you want to shape your hair firmly. These products give you the extra hold and extra shaping support necessary for precision styles. Modern gels are not sticky, and you can style your hair without the greasiness or flaking encountered with the gels that were available years ago.

Gels are versatile, providing anything from a natural to curly to a sleek, wet look, depending on how they are applied. For example, one leading manufacturer provides the following directions on the packaging of its gels:

For a natural look and extra volume, apply and spread evenly through the hair, then shape with a brush and dryer. For a sleek "wet" look, apply and comb through and shape, then air dry. For curly styles, apply evenly and generously, then make individual finger curls and air dry.

The versatility of these modern gels is due to the combinations of synthetic polymers they contain.

7

The Face: Basic Care and Common Problems

How to Cleanse the Face

What is the best method to cleanse the face? Some people claim soap and water is best, other claim that creams are best, and still others swear by liquid cleansers.

There is no one best method for cleansing the skin. Factors such as skin type, environment, and makeup are important considerations.

Furthermore, today there is a variety of cleansers to choose from. Bar cleansers may be either soap- or synthetic detergent-based and labeled for different kinds of skin: dry, oily, or combination. ("Soap and water" will be used here to refer to any soap- or detergent-based product.) They may also contain medications such as antibacterial agents or various types of abrasives. Liquid cleansers may be basically soap or detergent preparations that perform like soap, or they may be products that combine the attributes of soaps and creams. They may also contain antibacterial agents and/or exfoliants. A "cream" may be in the form of either a cream or a lotion.

Generally, soap-and-water cleansing (bar or liquid) satisfactorily cleanses the skin because soap and water efficiently removes most substances from the skin, including dirt, sweat, and other materials. But different types of skin may need different types of soap (or synthetic detergent) cleansers. Waterproof makeup is most easily removed with a cream, lotion, or liquid cleanser because it is oil- rather than water-soluble. In many instances, the most effective skin cleansing procedure consists of first using a cream or lotion cleanser to remove makeup and then gently washing the face with soap and water to remove the oily cream residue and other water-soluble materials. If the skin is excessively oily, a cream or lotion cleanser alone will leave the skin too oily. If the skin is excessively dry, frequent soap-and-water cleansing may strip too much oil and moisture from the skin, so it may be preferable to alternate between a cream cleanser and soap and water.

The various types of cream and liquid cleansers are discussed elsewhere in this chapter and in the following chapter.

Which Soap Is Best?

Does it matter which kind of soap you use to cleanse the face?

While we are bombarded with a variety of claims in ads for many kinds of soaps (and "soapless" cleansers, i.e., synthetic detergent-based bars and liquids), it is important to remember that the basic purpose is simply to cleanse the skin; most soaps will do this efficiently. Soap-and-water cleansing removes most substances from the skin surface, including contaminants such as dirt, oily soils, bacteria, and cosmetics, and natural skin products such as oils, dead cells, and sweat.

The choice of one soap over another depends primarily on personal preference, unless a physician has recommended a particular type of soap for a skin problem. The type of skin you have may influence your choice, as soaps for oily skin or medicated or abrasive soaps promoted for acne can be too harsh for dry skin. If your skin is oily, you might prefer a regular toilet soap or a soap formulated for oily skin over a superfatted soap, as the former generally are more efficient cleansers. Of course, you don't want to wash your face with an abrasive soap designed to remove dirt and grime from hands.

You should be able to find a soap that you like at the price you want to pay. Here's a brief description of the different types of cleansing bars and liquids to choose from.

Superfatted soaps contain more fatty materials such as cold cream, cocoa butter, neutral fats, or lanolin. Some people with dry skin find that superfatted soaps are less drying than regular toilet soaps. This may be because superfatting a soap actually makes it a less efficient cleanser, and this may be desirable if the skin is dry. But don't expect such a soap to take the place of a moisturizer after cleansing. While some superfatted soaps claim to "moisturize" the skin by leaving behind a residue of fat or cream, it is hardly likely that a cleansing agent can accomplish two diametrically opposed tasks in a single washing operation, by removing soil and debris from the skin and depositing a fat or cream on the skin. Other residue will stay behind too, and this residue may be irritating.

Soaps for oily skin generally contain more surfactant (soap or detergent) so they can do a more efficient job of removing excess oil from the skin. They may be too drying for other skin types, especially dry skin.

Transparent soaps, like superfatted soaps, contain more fat, as well as glycerin. Unfortunately, most transparent soaps do not lather as well and melt faster than regular soaps. They also tend to cost more, because the manufacture of transparent soaps is slower and most costly. No evidence exists that transparent soaps are milder than regular milled toilet soaps, but some people with dry, sensitive skin seem to prefer them.

Actually, many "soaps" today are actually synthetic detergent bars or liquids. Soaps are made from animal and vegetable fats, while synthetic detergent bars are made from petroleum derivatives. The primary advantage of detergents is that they do not interact with the minerals in hard water that form a soap scum. There is no evidence that detergent-based bars are harsher or milder than soap bars. But you shouldn't worry that using a detergent-based toilet bar is comparable to using laundry detergent on your face. The synthetic detergents used in skin cleansing products are mild.

All the liquid facial "soaps" contain at least some synthetic detergent, as it is not possible to formulate elegant liquid cleansers that are 100% soap. The choice of liquid over a bar is a matter of personal preference; they cleanse equally well.

Medicated and abrasive soaps intended for individuals with acne are discussed in Chapter 22. You can obtain more information on soaps by writing to the American Academy of Dermatology.

Astringents, Toners, Fresheners, and Clarifying Lotions

What's the difference between astringents, toners, fresheners, and clarifying lotions? Are they useful?

The nomenclature for this category of products has changed over the years, so it's difficult to define these products by name. The terms are used interchangeably to describe a type of product applied after cleansing to remove oil and other residue, for between-times cleansing, and sometimes just to "refresh" the skin. You must read the labels to determine what a particular product contains and its purpose.

A number of claims are made for these products—that they cleanse the skin, refine the texture, shrink pores, control oil, and help blemishes. In actuality, what most of these products do best is effectively remove oil from the skin's surface and produce a cool, refreshed feeling. None of these products will make your oil glands produce less oil; none of them permanently shrinks pores. The most they can do is temporarily make pores seem smaller by causing a swelling or slight irritation around the pores.

These products basically consist of water, alcohol, fragrance, and coloring agents. In addition to high levels of alcohol, products for oily skin will generally contain astringent ingredients such as witch hazel and menthol. They may contain resorcinol, which acts as a combination antiseptic, preservative, and astringent, and which may help to remove dead surface cells. Salicylic acid, which loosens dead cells on the skin surface, may also be included.

Products for either normal or dry skin usually contain mild cleansing ingredients as well as other ingredients that soothe the skin and aid in moisture retention. These products may contain low levels of alcohol, rose water, castor oil, glycerin, sodium borate, and allantoin.

Products for dry skin include very mild cleansers and skin-soothing ingredients. They contain little or no alcohol. These products are probably most effective at simply making the skin feel refreshed.

Individuals with dry skin should exercise caution in using any of these products, especially those that contain any alcohol or such ingredients as salicylic acid or resorcinol. Individuals with eczema or "sensitive skin" must also be cautious in the use of these products.

Care of an Oily Complexion

What type of skin care is recommended for an oily complexion?

The goal of caring for such skin is, of course, to minimize the degree of oiliness. Soap and water is the cheapest and most efficient means of cleansing oily skin. Cleansing creams or lotions will simply add to the oiliness. If you must use a cleansing cream to remove your makeup, follow it up with soap and water.

When washing is inconvenient, for example, at school or work, an astringent preparation or premoistened cleansing pads can be used. Most of these products contain alcohol to dissolve the oil; some contain surfactants to remove oil. Complexion brushes or abrasive soaps may irritate the skin if they are used too frequently.

Another convenient way to remove excess oil is to blot with special absorbent papers, which are available at pharmacies and cosmetic counters.

Wear water-based makeup rather than cream or oil-based products. These products are either oil-free or oil-in-water emulsions, as opposed to water-in-oil products. To determine whether a product is an oil-in-water emulsion, put a few drops in the palm. If it disappears without leaving a shiny film, it is oil-in-water and best for oily skin. If it seems not to dry at all or does so with a shiny film, it is water-in-oil and best for dry skin. Some "oil-free" products contain ingredients that are technically not oils but behave like oil, and therefore are not desirable for oily complexions. Water-based oil-free products usually have to be shaken before use as the pigments tend to settle in the bottom. Powder blushers and eyeshadow may be preferred. Use loose or dry, pressed powder.

The degree of oiliness of the skin varies with changes in sun and wind conditions, temperature, and emotions. When the weather is hot and humid and there is a lot of perspiration on the skin, it will appear more oily than when the weather is cold and dry. The skin's surface oil will spread out on a film of water in much the same way that a drop of motor oil spreads on the surface of a pond.

Summer and Oily Skin

My skin seems to get more oily in summer. What causes this?

Your skin doesn't really get more oily in summer. It just seems to because you naturally sweat more in summer, and as the oil and water mix they form an emulsion that spreads on the skin's surface and makes the skin look and feel more oily.

Combination Complexions

My cheeks and the area around my eyes are dry but my forehead, nose, and chin are oily. What type of skin care is recommended?

You probably have what is called a "combination complexion." There is a much greater concentration of active oil glands on the mid-forehead, nose, and chin than on the cheeks and temples and in the eye area. The central oily area is known as the "T-zone." Combination complexions, which are very common, present some problems in skin care and selection of cosmetics. The use of oily cosmetics make the center of the face too oily, while drying agents may irritate the sides of the face.

In addition, oiliness and dryness vary at different times of the year. The skin tends to be much drier during cold weather, when the humidity is lower. Even oily skin may become irritated or rough in the winter.

Proper care of combination skin requires a flexible skin-care regimen. Washing with a moderately drying soap two or three times a day will remove excess oil and decrease oiliness in the central area of your face. Excessive dryness on the sides of your cheeks and in the eye area may be relieved by a lubricating cream or lotion applied sparingly once or twice a day. Don't apply moisturizer to the oily areas, as this will simply exacerbate the oiliness. Between cleansings, a toner or astringent containing alcohol may be applied to the oily area.

You may have to experiment to find makeup that works. You will probably prefer makeup that is oil-free, water-based, or an oil-in-water emulsion rather than water-in-oil-based. You can apply a light, oil-in-water-based moisturizer to the dry areas prior to applying makeup. To determine whether makeup or moisturizer is oil-in-water, apply a few drops to the palm. If it disappears or dries quickly without leaving a shiny film, it is oil-in-water. If it doesn't seem to dry or does so with a shiny film, it is water-in-oil and best for dry skin. If you have to shake the product before use, it is probably water-based. If your cheeks are normal or dry, you can use cream blusher.

If your problem is serious or disturbing, you should consult a dermatologist.

Care of Dry Skin

What skin-care regimen is recommended for dry skin?

The key to caring for dry skin is to keep it moisturized. Replenishing the moisture in the skin will make it feel softer, smoother, and more comfortable.

Don't wash your face more than once a day with soap and water. Do this at bedtime, when you can remove makeup and the daily accumulation of grime. In the morning just splash the face with warm water. Always cleanse with warm rather than hot water.

If your face cannot tolerate daily soap-and-water cleansing, alternate with liquid, cream, or lotion cleansers. Avoid toners and fresheners that contain alcohol, which removes skin oils that act as a natural moisturizer.

After cleansing, apply a moisturizer to help retard moisture loss. During the day you may prefer a light oil-in-water emulsion that is non-greasy. At night, a heavier water-in-oil cream may be preferable. These products do not really add much moisture to the skin but they do help retard evaporation of moisture from the skin, allowing the skin to re-moisturize itself from within. They also make the skin feel softer, smoother, and more comfortable. (Moisturizers are discussed in detail in Chapter 8.)

Many factors influence the dryness of skin: age, geographical location, time of year, relative humidity in living and working quarters, and frequency of soap and detergent use. Individual variations under similar circumstances are probably due to hereditary differences.

If you live in a northern climate that becomes cold and dry in the winter, try to keep your environment humidified. Be sure to protect the face with a moisturizer when venturing out in cold, windy weather.

Finally, what you think is dry skin may not be helped by a dry-skin regimen: Flaking and scaling around the nose and chin may actually indicate excessively oily skin or seborrheic dermatitis rather than dry skin. If this is the case, application of greasy moisturizers and makeup will simply make your condition worse. These skin conditions are discussed elsewhere in this chapter.

Under-Makeup Color Correctors
or Toners

My complexion has become somewhat sallow as I've grown older. A friend suggested that I try one of the under-makeup color correctors. What do you think?

Under-makeup color correctors first became popular several years ago, and some cosmetic companies still include such a product in their lines.

Color correctors are applied as a film under regular makeup to even out skin tones. They can help brighten sallow complexions and even out irregular patches such as red blotches. They can also provide a tanned look. The effect resembles staining but is removed by soap and water or cleansing cream.

Under-makeup toners are available in several forms (liquids, creams, gels, and sticks) and colors. Green shades are intended to tone down florid (red) complexions; browns give a tanned look. Reddish, brown, or apricot colors are recommended for sallow complexions.

Consult the cosmetician in a local drug or department store about the shade and type of product that will be best for you.

Facial Masks

What benefits can one really expect from facial masks? Which are better, clay or peel-off masks?

Facial masks have been touted for centuries as providing special benefits such as minimizing wrinkles, improving texture, shrinking and unplugging pores, stimulating circulation, and smoothing and refreshing the skin. The *actual* benefits are few. Masks do not penetrate the skin, so the effects are superficial. They can help cleanse the skin and leave it looking and feeling smooth and refreshed for a few minutes to a few hours, but most of the benefits are psychological. As the mask dries, it produces a tightening, tingling feeling that makes us think something must be happening.

Traditional masks are based on absorbent materials such as purified earth and clay. As the water evaporates after application, the clay and earth harden to form a tight mask. When the mask is rinsed off after 15 to 20 minutes, oily materials, dirt, and dead surface cells trapped in the mask are also removed. These masks are intended mainly for oily skin but may also be used on normal or dry skin.

Newer innovations in masks include gel and peel-off masks. They are usually promoted for normal to dry skin. Gel masks, which are made with ingredients such as gum tragacanth, do not harden and are rinsed off after 10 to 15 minutes. Peel-off masks, made with polyvinyl alcohol or vinyl acetate, dry to form a sheer vinyl layer like a sheet of plastic. The layer is peeled off after 10 to 15 minutes.

Some "masks" for dry skin are not really masks at all but emollient, lubricating films that act in much the same way as moisturizers to soften and smooth the skin.

For the most part face masks are not harmful, although people with exceptionally dry skin may find regular masks irritating. People with oily skin may prefer clay masks. Whatever type of mask is used, it is important to carefully follow the manufacturer's directions for use. Don't apply a mask near the eyes unless the directions state that the mask may be applied to this area.

Exfoliating Products

How beneficial are exfoliating/sloughing products?

The outer layer of skin consists of dead cells that are constantly being sloughed off and replaced. In recent years cosmetic products to aid or speed up this sloughing action have become popular. The claims are that sloughing makes the complexion more radiant, youthful, and healthy-looking. Skin that has not had the benefit of exfoliation is supposedly dull-looking and old. The rationale behind these products is scientific evidence that, as skin ages, cell turnover slows down. These products are supposed to remove the dead cells that have failed to slough off on time.

These claims must be viewed with skepticism for a number of reasons. Normal skin does not need any aid in sloughing or exfoliating; it does this quite adequately itself. However, removal of the outer three to five layers of cells of the stratum corneum (the outer layer of skin), particularly if the skin is rough, makes light reflect more evenly and improves the skin's appearance. While it is true that as skin ages cell turnover is slowed down, the degree of sloughing that these products produce is not enough to produce visible results. Only more potent medical treatments can produce significant peeling or renewal (see Chapter 9 for more details).

Many products that are promoted as increasing exfoliation really do very little. Those that really work—such as abrasives—may be harmful. The abrasives exfoliate by mechanical means. Complexion brushes and abrasive pads fit in this category, as do products that contain mild abrasives such as apricot shells or synthetic particles.

The abrasive products may be of some benefit in acne, but abrasion or rough washing often makes acne worse. They should be used with caution on normal or, especially, dry skin, as they may be too irritating. The skin may become red, irritated, and overdry, and flake or peel. It's difficult for the average person to know how long and how often to use such products, to control the scrubbing pressure, and to adjust use according to changes in weather, water temperature, etc.

Makeup for Masking Birthmarks

Please provide information on special makeup that can be used to mask birthmarks.

There are a few brands of special cosmetics designed for camouflaging birthmarks. Most of these preparations are creams containing opaque masking agents such as titanium dioxide and zinc oxide. Pigments are added to provide a range of colors. They are waterproof and applied in a manner different from that for ordinary foundation makeups. They must be patted gently onto your skin and then set with a setting powder. You can then apply your regular makeup, or special makeup, over the camouflage.

Many brands of regular makeup include camouflage creams in their lines. These creams, some of which are available in lipstick-like applicators in several different shades, are helpful for concealing small areas. Many women use them to camouflage dark circles under the eyes and other minor cosmetic defects.

The keys to success in using any of these products include selecting the right shade to blend with the normal skin and learning the technique of application.

A couple of brands of cosmetics specially designed to mask birthmarks are available, but they have somewhat limited distribution. A dermatologist can advise you about availability of these products or recommend other products that have proved helpful. He may also be able to recommend a good makeup artist who can teach you how to skillfully apply cosmetics. A dermatologist can also inform you about treatments by which certain types of birthmarks can be removed or made less noticeable (see Chapter 26 for information on common birthmarks).

Products to Lighten Dark Complexions

What's your opinion of creams advertised to lighten and brighten dark skin? I have blotchy skin that I would like to even out, or "lighten and brighten," as the ads claim.

If your skin is normally blotchy—that is, the pigmentation is just uneven—you probably will not be satisfied with the results obtained from such creams. At present, there is no readily available product that will safely, simply, and effectively lighten normal skin.

These products generally contain hydroquinone as the bleaching agent. Hydroquinone is somewhat effective when used to treat excess pigmentation caused by disease or injury. It is less effective as a depigmenting agent on normal skin. Results also depend on concentration of the hydroquinone in the product and on exposure to sun.

The response of normal black skin to hydroquinone treatment for depigmentation depends on the amount and depth of the pigment in the skin. Lighter black skin is partly depigmented, while no depigmentation of darker skin is observed. After treatment is stopped, repigmentation almost always occurs.

Many people who use "skin-tone creams" are really using them for their emollient or skin-softening effects. Such effects can easily be obtained with simple, non-medicated moisturizers.

Which Cosmetic Brand Is Best?

There are so many different brands of cosmetics that I don't know which one is best. Are expensive, department-store brands better than those in drugstores? Any advice would be welcome.

No one brand of cosmetics is best. Most are very similar. Selection of one brand over another usually depends solely on personal preference for such characteristics as shade, scent, texture, ease of use, and package design and presentation.

Price does not necessarily indicate quality in cosmetics. Some low-priced products have proven, over years of satisfactory use, to compare favorably with similar but more expensive products.

Manufacturers of brand-name products depend on repeat sales for success, so they are going to make the products as trouble-free as possible to help gain wide acceptance.

If you don't need any advice on selecting shades and types of cosmetics or on technique of application, you may prefer to purchase your products at a drugstore. If you would like such assistance, you may prefer to spend more and shop at a department store where there usually are trained cosmetic sales personnel to help you. Others prefer to buy their products at home from one of the companies that distribute directly through trained salespersons. The channel of distribution does not reflect quality.

Use the products you like, whether they are inexpensive or expensive. Don't let yourself be pushed into buying products that you will never use, or don't know how to use properly. Many women (and men) have drawers full of such products.

Chapped Lips

I'm plagued with chapped lips all winter. What causes them? What can I do to avoid them?

Chapped lips occur from repeated wetting and drying. They are more common in the winter when the cold, dry, windy weather dries out the lips. When the lips (or any other skin area) lose too much moisture, the outer cell layers become rough, dry, and inflexible. Painful cracks may develop.

To minimize the chapping, avoid licking the lips. Use a lip protector, such as a moisturizer or lipstick. Moisturizers are available as clear waxy ointments, creams, or sticks. Many contain sunscreens. Apply the moisturizer regularly and frequently, whenever the lips feel dry and at bedtime, especially if you have a cold or are a mouth breather.

If chapped lips persist, you may want to consult a dermatologist. Sometimes chapped lips are caused by eczema or allergic contact dermatitis.

Milia

I have little hard knots under my skin that I thought were whiteheads but my dermatologist says they are milia. What are milia?

Milia are small epithelial cysts that clinically resemble white-heads. They are hard, painless, and stationary, and generally remain white. Milia may occur spontaneously (usually around the eyes), after abrasive injury to the skin and after blisters.

If only a few milia are present, your doctor may just nick them at the top with a fine scalpel or needle and express the contents. If they are numerous, electrosurgery, dermabrasion, or peeling may be necessary.

Enlarged Pores

What can I do to get rid of the enlarged pores on my face? They are especially large on my nose.

An enlarged pore is the opening of a follicle that usually has a tiny, invisible hair and large, active sebaceous (oil) glands. Enlarged pores are most obvious on the nose, forehead, and inner aspects of the cheeks and chin, where the oil glands are concentrated. Oily skin and acne often accompany enlarged pores.

Nothing can change the size of enlarged pores or prevent more from developing, so don't believe claims that any product or treatment will "shrink" them.

You can temporarily improve the appearance of enlarged pores with cosmetics. Astringent preparations, which contain ingredients such as witch hazel and alcohol, may make pores less obvious for a short time. They irritate the surrounding skin so that it swells slightly around the pores. Inflammation, from sunburn, for example, may cause swelling (edema) of the skin, making pores appear smaller for a short period. When carefully selected and applied, makeup can help conceal enlarged pores. You may have to try several different makeup bases to find the one best suited for your skin.

Melasma, The Mask of Pregnancy

I'm pregnant, and I've developed brownish patches on my face. Is this discoloration permanent? What can be done for it?

Many pregnant women develop brownish patches on their cheeks or forehead or around the eyes. The medical terms for this problem are *melasma* and *chloasma*, but it is commonly called "the mask of pregnancy." It results from an increase of pigment and is most common in brunettes, women of Mediterranean descent, and those who spend a lot of time in the sun.

Because it is related to hormonal changes, melasma may also occur in women who are taking birth control pills. Melasma due to pregnancy should fade gradually within several months after childbirth. Melasma caused by birth control pills may be more persistent.

Sun intensifies melasma, so you should wear a sunscreen (SPF 15 or more) that blocks both UVB and UVA radiation whenever you are out in the sun. These products will not stop the increase in pigment but are helpful in minimizing the sun's effects. You can conceal the discoloration with a masking cream worn under your makeup. Your doctor may prescribe a bleaching preparation containing hydroquinone to help fade the pigmentation. These products are quite effective for some individuals but not for others. They generally must be used for many months to achieve results.

Seborrheic Dermatitis on the Face

I have red, scaling areas on my face that I thought were due to dry skin, but my dermatologist says it's seborrheic dermatitis associated with excess oiliness. I would appreciate more information on this skin problem.

Seborrheic dermatitis is one of the most common skin disorders seen by dermatologists. It is mainly a cosmetic problem and usually can be easily treated.

In this chronic disorder, inflammation occurs in the skin areas that have the greatest number of sebaceous (oil) glands. The affected skin is not only oily but inflamed (red) and covered with whitish or yellowish greasy scales. There may also be mild burning or itching. Common sites for seborrheic dermatitis include the forehead, mid-face, the sides of the nose and the chin (the "T-zone"), eyebrows and eyelids, and behind and inside the ears. (Other common sites are the scalp and, in men, the chest.)

The cause is unknown. Infants with a predisposition toward seborrheic dermatitis will have cradle cap and perhaps a tendency to develop severe diaper rash. Children and adolescents generally show no characteristics other than dandruff. Seborrheic dermatitis becomes evident in adulthood, although sometimes not until late in life. Adults with chronic neurological conditions (for example, Parkinson's disease) often have seborrheic dermatitis, as do some patients recovering from stressful medical situations such as heart attacks. Others with seborrheic dermatitis are perfectly healthy.

There is no way to prevent or cure seborrheic dermatitis, but it can be controlled. Washing the face two or three times a day with a moderately drying soap usually controls facial oiliness. Your dermatologist can prescribe a topical medication to control redness and scaling. (See Chapter 2 for information on controlling seborrheic dermatitis of the scalp, which usually accompanies facial seborrheic dermatitis.) You can obtain more information on seborrheic dermatitis from the American Academy of Dermatology.

Rosacea

My face is red and has acne-like blemishes. My doctors say I have rosacea. What causes this problem? What treatment is recommended?

Rosacea is a chronic disease that affects men and women in their thirties, forties, and fifties. It is characterized by redness of the central area of the face due to dilation of small blood vessels (telangiectasia). The dilation may be fleeting or long-lasting. The condition is sometimes called acne rosacea because acne-like blemishes are the main symptom of the disorder. However, in rosacea blackheads and whiteheads are not present; this can help the dermatologist to distinguish it from common acne.

Besides the red facial flushing and blemishes, the oil glands on the nose may be enlarged, resulting in a condition known as rhinophyma (see the following question and answer).

Rosacea is a complex problem, the cause of which remains unknown. Emotional stress, extremes of temperature, alcohol, hot beverages, and products containing sorbic acid, a food preservative, can aggravate the condition. You should leave treatment in the hands of your dermatologist, who will consider such factors as the stage and severity of the disease and your age. Antibiotics may be prescribed. Drying and antiseptic—as well as soothing—local preparations may be prescribed. Any blemishes will be treated like those in a regular case of acne. The dilated blood vessels and overgrown sebaceous glands can also be treated.

Rhinophyma

I've developed a big, red, lumpy, bumpy nose that looks like W. C. Fields' nose. But I don't even drink. What causes this? Can it be treated?

You probably have a condition known as rhinophyma, a severe form of rosacea (see the previous question and answer). The lower half of the nose becomes red and bumpy because of an overgrowth of sebaceous glands and dilated blood vessels. Other midline facial areas may be similarly involved. The condition primarily affects middle-aged and older men. The overgrowth of the nose may at times be quite large and present a severe cosmetic and social defect.

Rhinophyma is chronic but treatable. Various topical and internal medications may be helpful in the early stages. Large broken blood vessels can be destroyed by electrocoagulation. In advanced stages, the best treatment for rhinophyma is surgery. Under local, or sometimes general, anesthesia, the nose can be reshaped by removing superfluous tissue. Dermabrasion, electrosurgery, or laser surgery may be used. Consult a dermatologist about treatment.

Enlarged Blood Vessels on the Face

I've developed spidery, enlarged blood vessels on my face. What causes this, and what treatment is available?

Enlarged blood vessels are referred to as *telangiectases*. The many possible causes include heredity, overexposure to sunlight, liver damage, pregnancy, and rosacea (see earlier discussion in this chapter). Injuries, and even a mosquito bite, can cause telangiectases. You would have to consult a physician for an accurate diagnosis of your particular case.

Further telangiectasia can be prevented in some instances, depending on the cause of the condition. In general, exposure to cold, wind, sun and heat; rapid changes in temperature; and very hot or highly spiced foods and beverages should be avoided.

Some isolated telangiectases may disappear spontaneously. They can sometimes be concealed with cosmetic cover creams. Various medical treatments are also effective; your physician can advise you about them.

Bags Under the Eyes

What causes bags under the eyes?

Pouching and drooping skin under the eyes is primarily due to heredity and usually occurs with advancing age although it may occur earlier. Normally, the skin in this area is delicate and loosely attached. As a person grows older, some underlying muscles and tissues degenerate, and the lower lids tend to fall in folds. Underlying fat pushes through weakened muscles, causing the baggy tissue to balloon out.

When bags are extreme, they may constitute a disfigurement that is a social and economic handicap, especially in a young person. Cosmetics offer little or no help.

Plastic surgery is the only method that will improve this condition. The operation is referred to as *blepharoplasty.* It can be done either in an outpatient surgical clinic or in a hospital. Swelling and discoloration generally subside within 2 weeks, and scars are usually well camouflaged.

You should consult a physician experienced in plastic surgery for specific details.

Dark Circles Under the Eyes

What causes dark circles under eyes? I get plenty of sleep but still have this problem.

Dark circles under the eyes are usually unrelated to physical disease or the amount of sleep you get; the condition depends on several anatomical factors and may reflect a family trait. The skin of the eyelids is thin and contains little fatty tissue. Blood that passes through large veins close to the surface shows through the skin, producing a bluish-black tint. Also, in time, there may be some leakage of blood, as with varicose veins on the lower legs.

Dark circles are accentuated when one is tired and pale, during menstruation, and in the latter part of pregnancy. With aging the discoloration may become more obvious and permanent.

The dark circles can usually be concealed with the camouflage creams that many cosmetic companies include in their makeup lines. Seek the advice of the cosmetic salesperson on shade and technique of application. Those who wear glasses may find that tinted lenses will help make dark circles under their eyes less noticeable.

Fatty Deposits on the Eyelids

I've developed yellowish fatty deposits on my upper eyelids. Does this indicate a medical problem? Can they be removed?

Raised, soft, yellowish deposits of fat on the eyelids usually represent cholesterol deposits known as *xanthelasmas*. They are more common on the upper eyelids than the lower, but may appear on both. About one-fourth to one-half of the individuals with xanthelasmas have elevated blood cholesterol levels. This may be familial.

You should consult your physician to determine whether your problem is related to elevated blood cholesterol levels that may require treatment.

The fatty deposits can be removed by various techniques, including chemical application of trichloroacetic acid, electrosurgery, cryosurgery, or scissor excision. The cosmetic results after any of the methods are usually excellent, but recurrences are common. You should leave the choice of treatment up to your physician.

Waterproof Eye Makeup

Is there any eye makeup that is really waterproof? Is it best to use eye-makeup remover or will cleansing cream or soap and water do as good a job?

It is doubtful that any eye makeup is completely waterproof. However, products advertised as waterproof generally do remain in place longer than others.

Many waterproof eye cosmetics are, in the simplest terms, composed of either a pigmented waxy base dissolved in a volatile solvent or a pigment suspended in a gum or resin solution.

There are two categories of waterproof cosmetics: 1) those that resist tears, moisture in the air, and perspiration and 2) those that resist all of these plus ordinary soap and water. The second type requires some other means of removal. Products that contain a solvent such as mineral oil or a similar oil will work well. Most facial cleansing creams, oils, and lotions, as well as most eye-makeup removers, contain one or more of these solvents as basic ingredients, so any of these products will effectively remove most waterproof eye makeup. Individuals who wear contact lenses may prefer a non-oily makeup remover to creams or oils, as the latter can more easily get on lenses and blur vision.

Mascara for Contact Lens Wearers

I wear contact lenses. Should I use one of the special mascaras that are promoted for contact lens wearers? How do these products differ from regular mascara?

Mascara is generally a combination of soap, wax, or liquid and pigments designed to color the eyelashes. It is available in cream and liquid forms. Cream mascara, an aqueous emulsion, comes in a tube and is applied with a brush. Liquid mascara is similar to the cream type, but is usually packaged in a hard cylinder with a built-in brush applicator. It is also more water-resistant than cake mascara. Lash-extender mascara is liquid mascara with tiny synthetic fibers added. As the liquid evaporates, the fibers adhere to the wet lashes, making them appear thicker and longer.

People who wear contact lenses are advised to avoid lash-extender mascara because the fibers may get in the eye, causing irritation under the lens. The products promoted especially for contact lens wearers are liquid mascaras that do not contain lash-extender fibers. They may also contain a different preservative from that in regular mascara. Those who wear contact lenses may develop a sensitivity to phenylmercuric acid (PMA), a preservative used in other eye products, because some lens-cleaning solutions contain this ingredient. Mascaras labeled as safe for contact lens wearers, then, should not contain PMA. (Most products promoted for contact lens wearers are ophthalmologist-tested.)

Contact lenses should be inserted before the application of eye makeup and removed before makeup is removed.

See the following discussion for precautions for all people who wear eye makeup such as mascara and eyeliner.

Eye Makeup Precautions

Why is it harmful to borrow eye makeup? I thought the products contain preservatives to protect against infection. Are there any other precautions that should be observed?

It is not advisable to borrow eye makeup because you may pick up an eye infection. For instance, several years ago there was an epidemic of an eye infection called trachoma among schoolgirls borrowing eyeliner pencils.

Eye makeup, and other cosmetics, do contain preservatives to minimize the danger of contamination; however, the preservatives require a period of time between uses to do their job. The concentration of the preservative used is adjusted for chemical as well as microbiological safety, according to normal use patterns for such products. Only a very strong preservative in high concentrations could maintain a cosmetic product at near sterile levels, especially shortly after use. Since such strong preservatives in the necessary concentrations pose safety problems of a different type, their use in eye cosmetics is not desirable. So, to avoid infections, don't borrow or lend eye cosmetics; by doing so you defeat the built-in safeguards.

Eye makeup should not be subjected to excessive heat, for example, by placing it on a radiator or in a glove compartment. Bacterial contamination may occur from many sources. Therefore: 1) nothing extraneous should be placed in or on an eye product; 2) never dilute your eye makeup with anything, including water; 3) keep the container closed when not in use; 4) do not purchase refills that require re-use of the original brush or applicator; 5) don't use saliva to wet cake mascara or eyeliner.

Eyeliner should not be extended to the canthus (the area where the upper and lower lids meet) because the material can easily be carried into the eye by the moisture in this region. Eyeliner should also not be applied on the eyelid between the eyelashes and the ball of the eye.

Finally, remember that special care must be taken in the application of eye makeup. Apply the makeup at home, not in an automobile or any other moving vehicle. Serious inflammation of the eye has occurred following a scratch on the cornea caused by an applicator brush accidently hitting the eye.

Permanent Eyeliner

What is your opinion of permanent eyeliners? What does this technique involve? Is it safe?

The technique by which a permanent "eyeliner" is placed on the upper (and sometimes lower) eyelids is called permanent micropigmentation surgery. It is a variation of tattooing that involves implanting metallic oxide pigments along the upper and lower lashes. The depth of color achieved depends on the application time and the use of lighteners, such as talc or titanium dioxide, added to the pigment. The procedure, which can be performed in a physician's office, is rather new—it is performed by only a limited number of plastic surgeons and dermatologists. All the pros and cons of this technique have yet to be evaluated.

Some physicians have reservations about micropigmentation surgery. One potential problem is delayed hypersensitive reactions to the pigment itself or to the lighteners. This may be avoided by spot testing a few months prior to applying the full tattoo, although a negative spot test does not rule out the possibility of a reaction since a reaction may develop many months later. Another problem with such surgery is that the eyeliner color may begin to look harsh as the individual ages and skin and hair color naturally fade.

On the other hand, permanent eyeliner may be a boon to those who are unable to wear regular eyeliner because of allergic sensitivity or who lack the manual dexterity to apply regular eyeliner.

8

Facial Creams and Other Facial Products

Cold Creams and Cleansing Creams

Does it matter whether I use a cold cream or a cleansing cream to cleanse my skin?

Not really. It's a matter of personal preference. Cold cream is the prototype of all cleansing and emollient creams and lotions. Prior to its development, people had to rely on plain animal and vegetable oils to cleanse and lubricate the skin.

The first cold cream was a mixture of oil, water, beeswax, and rose petals. The beeswax acted as an emulsifier to keep the oil and water mixed; rose petals provided fragrance. When applied to the skin for cleansing, the oil picked up and suspended the dirt, oil, and other skin debris so it could be wiped off. If left on the skin, it acted as a lubricant or emollient (moisturizer). The product was called a "cold" cream because it felt cooling as the water evaporated.

Modern cold creams, cleansing creams, and emollient creams bear little resemblance to the original, crude cold cream, although the basic formula of all modern creams is a variation of the original cold cream formula: an oil-and-water emulsion. There is now an infinite variety of creams, lotions, and mousses, with many different textures, consistencies, colors, smells, and cleansing qualities. For example, a product may be formulated so that it can be rinsed from the skin rather than wiped off. Surfactants are often added to increase the cleansing qualities and aid removal. Products formulated to remove heavy theatrical make-up may contain more oils. Products for oily skin are modified to remove more of the natural oils and fats from the skin, whereas creams formulated for dry skin may contain ingredients to reduce the products' oil-removing properties and/or to replace oils removed in the cleansing process.

Cold creams are generally heavier; they produce more drag on the skin than cleansing creams. Some women prefer the lighter feel of cleansing creams.

Cream Versus Soap and Water for Cleansing

Do cleansing creams adequately clean the skin or should I also wash my face with soap and water?

That depends on what you are trying to remove from the skin. Creams and lotions are better for removing makeup, especially if it is waterproof (eye makeup, for example) but other materials are removed more thoroughly by soap and water.

The best method of cleansing also depends to some degree on your skin type. Individuals with oily skin should follow cream cleansing with soap and water to remove the cream's oily residue. Individuals with extremely dry skin may find daily soap-and-water cleansing too drying. Probably the best all-around cleansing procedure for those who wear makeup is a combination of cream and soap-and-water cleansing. First remove makeup with cleansing cream or lotion, then wash the skin with soap and water to remove the oily residue and other materials left on the skin. (If the skin feels too dry after cleansing, apply a moisturizer.)

If you wear eye makeup and do not want to use a cleansing cream or lotion, you can use an eye-makeup remover followed by soap and water. (Eye-makeup removers are discussed at the end of this chapter.)

Emollient, Lubricating, and Moisturizing Creams

What's the difference between lubricating, emollient, and moisturizing creams? It's very confusing. How can I know what kind of cream I should use?

You are not alone in your confusion. Drugstore and department store shelves are filled with hundreds of products that fit in the broad moisturizer/emollient category. Magazines are stuffed with ads touting "unique" benefits to be derived from different products. There are eye, throat, and facial creams, lotions, and mousses.

These products are all variations on a theme. They all perform basically the same function even though the texture, consistency, color, smell, price, and packaging differ. "Moisturizers" counteract the stiffness of the outer regions of the stratum corneum (the outer portion of the epidermis) and make it more pliable and less prone to crack, making the surface feel softer and smoother. They achieve these results primarily by slowing down the loss of moisture from the skin by depositing a film of oil that helps retard evaporation of moisture. Some products contain moisture-binding or hydrating ingredients that enable them to increase the skin's moisture level without being heavy and occlusive.

The distinctions between the terms *moisturizer, emollient,* and *lubricant* have more to do with marketing than with science. Consumers and marketing people like *moisturizer* because it suggests that the product actually changes the skin. Women mistakenly associate dryness with aging skin; moist skin is supposed to be beautiful and youthful. Consumers generally think of an emollient as simply a skin softener; the term is thus less popular as a product description.

Moisturizing/emollient products are formulated as either oil-in-water (O/W) or water-in-oil (W/O) emulsions. W/O emulsions contain more oil, are heavier, and generally provide longer-lasting effects, so they are often used for products such as night creams. Most lighter, less greasy products such as daytime moisturizers and lotions are O/W emulsions.

Animal, vegetable, mineral, and synthetic oils may be used in moisturizers. Some products that contain synthetic oils or ingredients that perform the same function as oils claim to be "oil-free." These synthetic ingredients include high-molecular-weight sugars and volatile silicones.

Moisturizers are often promoted as containing special ingredients that penetrate the skin to enhance the moisturizing effects, speed cell renewal, improve microcirculation, and retard aging. You will find a discussion of many of these and other ingredients, as well as of various types of creams, elsewhere in this chapter.

The most important question regarding moisturizers may be

whether you need one. If your skin is excessively oily, you really don't need to use any type of moisturizing cream. And just because your skin is flaking does not mean that it is dry; flaking can occur with seborrheic dermatitis, a condition associated with oily skin. If your skin is indeed dry, then you should select a moisturizing product that you like and can afford. If your skin is *very* dry, you will probably prefer a cream to a lotion.

How to Apply Facial Creams

Does it matter how I apply a moisturizing cream? The cosmetic salesperson said I must apply it with upward and outward strokes to prevent sagging skin.

It doesn't matter how you apply a cream as long as you do it gently. You don't want to irritate the skin by rubbing it too vigorously.

Skin sags for reasons that have nothing to do with how you apply your moisturizer. Aging, sun damage, gravity, loss of muscle tone, genetic predisposition, and other factors are the villains, not the method of application of makeup or creams.

The Skin's Natural Moisturizing Factor

Some creams claim to contain the skin's natural moisturizing factor and therefore to be better. What does this mean? Are these creams really better?

The skin's natural moisturizing factor (NMF) has been the object of research for years. It appears that the skin may have such a factor, but its exact nature is unknown. NMF is now considered mainly a marketing gimmick.

Some investigators believe that lipids (fats) that are found between the cells of the stratum corneum (outer layer of the epidermis) play a significant role in helping the skin maintain adequate moisture and therefore are part of the NMF. It is also thought that these lipids are lost from the stratum corneum through various environmental exposures, including exposure to soap and water and other solvents.

Cosmetic ingredients that have been touted as achieving the effects of the skin's NMF include urea, lactic acid, and phospholipids. The use of urea in cosmetic products is based on its ability to attract and hold water. Theoretically it diffuses into the stratum corneum, where it supposedly allows water to be transported more easily into the stratum corneum. The use of lactic acid in emollient products is based on research that indicates that the stratum corneum is more pliable when it absorbs lactic acid. Phospholipids are discussed in the following question and answer.

Phospholipids in Creams

What do phospholipids do in moisturizers? Are they better for dry skin? Do they help to retard aging?

Phospholipids are part of the lipids (fats) that surround the cells in the stratum corneum, as discussed in the previous question and answer on the skin's natural moisturizing factor.

When certain lipids in the skin are decreased, the stratum corneum's barrier function is impaired and too much moisture may escape from the skin, causing it to become rough and dry. It is claimed that phospholipids added to moisturizers penetrate into the stratum corneum and act in much the same way that the skin's natural fats do in helping to hold moisture in the skin.

Whether the addition of phospholipids to emollient creams makes them more suitable for dry skin is still open to debate. However, some dermatologists believe that their patients seem to do better when such products are used. Others do not find them to be superior. Dermatologists are unified, however, in their opinion that adding phospholipids to creams will not help to reverse the effects of aging on the skin.

Cell Renewal Creams

What is your opinion of products that claim to increase the rate of cell turnover or aid cell renewal? I understand that as the skin ages the rate of cell turnover slows down and this makes the skin look older.

Cell renewal or cell turnover refers to the time required for newly formed cells to move from the base of the epidermis, where they are formed, to the surface, where they are sloughed off. It takes about a month for a cell to turn over in young skin (about 15 days to travel from the base of the epidermis to the stratum corneum, the dead outer layer of the skin, and about 15 days to move from the base of the stratum corneum to the surface). It may take almost twice as long for this turnover to occur in elderly skin.

It's claimed that the longer the process takes, the more apt the skin is to develop a dull, drab appearance. There are also claims that this slower cell transit can adversely affect the barrier function of the stratum corneum so the skin loses moisture more rapidly and is thus more likely to become overly dry.

Advertising and packaging claims for cell renewal products refer to tests that prove that a particular product increases the rate of cell turnover. The fact is, however, that application of many moisturizers will increase the rate of cell turnover. More important to the consumer is the question of whether the increase in the rate of cell turnover will produce any visible difference in the skin, by, for example, smoothing out wrinkles. This is very doubtful. Most agents that increase cell turnover improve the appearance of dry skin simply through their moisturizing qualities.

Creams to Improve Microcirculation

Some creams claim to improve the microcirculation of the skin and thus make it more youthful-looking. Is this possible, or desirable?

Some cosmetic manufacturers claim that improving the circulation of the small vessels near the skin surface augments the blood flow, ultimately feeding the skin with more oxygen and nutrients. Various techniques have established that some products do indeed temporarily increase the microcirculation of the skin. But improving the blood flow will do no more than give a "healthy glow" to washed-out, pale skin (although this alone might be considered an adequate enhancement of physical appearance). There is no good, objective, scientific evidence that supplying the skin with more oxygen and nutrients will make aged skin look younger. Of course, this does not stop creative copywriters from implying that it will.

Hormone Creams

Are hormone creams effective in retarding or reversing aging? I don't see them advertised anymore.

Hormone creams are classified as drugs by the FDA because their manufacturers maintain that they affect the structure and function of the skin (i.e., reverse the changes that aging causes in the skin). Thus, the claims made for these products must be shown to be true. Cosmetics must meet no such criteria.

An expert advisory panel that reviewed hormone creams for efficacy reported:

> The medical literature indicates that the topical application of hormone-containing drug products may affect the cellular structure of the skin but these changes are observable only through a microscope. ... The Panel believes that it is possible that the mild dermal edema, which was difficult to demonstrate histologically, may be produced equally well by a moisturizing cream which does not contain hormones. ... The Panel further concludes that there is no evidence that using a hormone-containing drug product at the levels which are safe for over-the-counter (non-prescription) use will do anything more than the cream containing the vehicle alone. Therefore, the Panel concludes that these products are ineffective for OTC drug use.

Since the FDA does not consider these products to be effective, they are not supposed to be sold any longer. Most major manufacturers have complied with the FDA recommendation; that's why you haven't seen hormone creams advertised lately. You will obtain just as good a result from using a moisturizing product that does not contain hormones, and will probably save money too.

The administration of estrogen to postmenopausal women to improve skin appearance, among other effects, should not be confused with the application of hormone creams. Evidence is accumulating that estrogen replacement therapy may have a significant effect on the skin.

Collagen and Elastin in Cosmetic Creams

I understand that the skin is composed primarily of collagen and elastin, which is damaged with aging, so creams that contain these ingredients are the best. Is this true?

Your statement is, at best, only partially correct. The inner layer of the skin, the dermis, is composed mainly of collagen and elastin. Collagen, a protein, is a primary constituent of all connective tissue, including the dermis. It provides structure to the dermis and is the major source of the skin's strength. Elastin, the other major component of the dermis, forms fibers that give skin its elasticity. When the elastic fibers are in good condition, the skin is able to stretch and then return to its normal condition. You are able to gain and lose weight without the skin sagging. When elastin fibers become damaged or frayed, the skin loses this stretchability and will sag instead of snapping back, and wrinkles will appear.

Overexposure to the sun (and, to a lesser degree, aging) produces changes in the collagen and elastic fibers that cause the skin to sag and become wrinkled and less flexible.

There is some evidence that adding collagen may improve the moisturizing qualities of a product and provide a cosmetic "feel" that consumers seem to prefer. But manufacturers imply that collagen and/or elastin in cosmetic products will rejuvenate or replace the damaged collagen and elastin, making the skin look younger. This is impossible. Neither of these ingredients can penetrate the skin because their molecules are too large. Furthermore, the collagen and elastin incorporated into these products are either derived from animal sources or synthetic, so they cannot replace the skin's collagen and elastin, and certainly will not rejuvenate the skin.

Liposomes in Cosmetic Creams

What are liposomes? What special benefits do they provide in moisturizing creams? Will liposomes really help rejuvenate the skin?

Liposomes are one of the new "wonder" ingredients being added to moisturizing creams to support anti-aging claims. The theory behind liposomes mixes some science with a lot of "puffery" or conjecture.

Liposomes are being investigated in medicine as delivery systems to target drugs in order to minimize adverse effects. In cosmetics, liposomes ostensibly target ingredients right to the cells so that the cells begin to "act young" again. Liposomes are supposed to enable ingredients to penetrate down between the cell layers of the stratum corneum, the outer layer of the skin, to help the skin retain more moisture. There are also claims that when cosmetic ingredients such as collagen and elastin are encapsulated into liposomes, the ingredients can penetrate not only the stratum corneum but the whole epidermis, to reach the dermis where human collagen and elastin are located. There the collagen and elastin in the liposomes will supposedly be able to rejuvenate or replace the skin's collagen and elastin.

Medical experts are skeptical. Molecules of collagen and elastin are too large to penetrate the skin, and it is not clear how encapsulating the molecules in liposomes will shrink them. Experts question whether liposomes can indeed penetrate the skin and, even if they can, whether the ingredients in the liposomes can have any effect on the skin's cells, especially that of making the cells "young" again. Dermatologists who have done research on aging agree that the aging process is very complex, with many unknowns, but they seriously doubt the claims being made for the rejuvenating qualities of liposomes.

Of course, by the time you read this, liposomes will probably have been replaced by some new "wonder" ingredient.

Hyaluronic Acid and Mucopolysaccharides in Creams and Lotions

Many cosmetic creams now list hyaluronic acid and mucopolysaccharides as ingredients. What are these things? What special benefits do they provide?

Mucopolysaccharides are components of the dermis, the inner layer of the skin. The two primary components of the dermis are collagen and elastin, as discussed earlier. Mucopolysaccharides are gel-like substances that surround the collagen and elastin fibers. About 70% of the mucopolysaccharides in skin are hyaluronic acid.

Just exactly what special benefits these ingredients are supposed to provide to the skin is not clear. They may act as moisture-binding agents to help attract and hold moisture. However, since they don't penetrate the skin, they have no effect on the mucopolysaccharides in the dermis.

One form of hyaluronic acid that is promoted by cosmetic manufacturers is supposed to be very hydrophyllic (water-attracting) and therefore useful in moisturizers—but equally good moisturization can be obtained with less expensive ingredients. You will probably pay a premium price for a cream that contains hyaluronic acid because it costs the manufacturer more. But just because it costs more does not mean that it is better. (Hyaluronic acid has been used as an inert gel in eye surgery, but this use has nothing to do with its presumed benefit as a cosmetic ingredient. Any correlation is misleading.)

Glycerin in Creams

I've heard conflicting stories about glycerin. Some say it helps to moisturize the skin, while others say it is actually drying because it draws moisture from the skin. What are the facts?

The fact is that glycerin is a beneficial ingredient in creams and lotions because it is a humectant, that is, it attracts moisture. It helps keep the product moist and attracts moisture to the upper layers of skin where it's needed to relieve dry skin. It also makes products spread better. A formulation known as glycerin and rose water is one of the classic emollients/moisturizers. It was used by our great-grandmothers and is still used today.

If you apply straight 100% glycerin to the skin, it might be drying because of its humectant qualities, but the concentration of glycerin in creams is never higher than 50%.

Glycerin is perfectly safe. It is used in medications that are taken internally as well as in products applied to the skin.

Mineral Oil in Creams

Is it true that mineral oil can be absorbed through the skin and cause cancer, so you shouldn't use any cosmetic creams that contain mineral oil?

Mineral oil is a perfectly safe cosmetic ingredient. It is not absorbed by the skin and won't cause cancer. If mineral oil were harmful, you wouldn't be able to buy it for internal use as a laxative/lubricant. The misconception that mineral oil is carcinogenic evidently arose from the fact that it is derived from petroleum, and certain petroleum derivatives are carcinogens.

Mineral oil is widely used in creams and lotions because it is inexpensive and an excellent emollient. The only drawback is that it is rather greasy. Packaging and advertising for products that do not contain mineral oil will sometimes highlight this fact as a way of indicating that the product is not greasy.

The only cosmetic use to which you shouldn't put pure mineral oil is as a suntan oil. It is not a sunscreen, and so it won't help prevent sunburning; all it will do is lubricate the skin.

Vitamin A in Creams

Is it true that creams that contain vitamin A may be as effective as vitamin A acid for making skin look younger?

Cosmetic creams that contain plain vitamin A will not have the same effects on the skin as topical treatment with vitamin A acid.

Some cosmetic creams and lotions contain derivatives of vitamin A called retinyl esters, such as retinol palmitate. These ingredients are converted into vitamin A acid when applied to the skin. It is questionable, though, whether the amount of retinyl ester converted into vitamin A acid is enough to provide the therapeutic effects provided by topical vitamin A acid.

You should view with skepticism all anti-aging claims for cosmetic creams.

Petroleum Jelly as a Moisturizer

I heard that plain old petroleum jelly works just as well as those expensive creams to relieve dry skin. Is this true?

It certainly is. The only problem is that you may find petroleum jelly (petrolatum) less cosmetically acceptable than a regular moisturizer because it is rather thick and greasy and doesn't spread easily over large areas.

Petrolatum has been used for over 100 years. It leaves a heavy occlusive film on the skin that acts as a barrier to loss of moisture and to irritation from environmental contacts. It is such an effective barrier that it is considered a superior moisturizer. Petrolatum is often a key ingredient in emollient creams and lotions because it is so effective in relieving the symptoms of dry skin. It's also used as a soothing treatment for minor skin irritations. Mothers sometimes apply it to the diaper area to help prevent diaper rash.

Eye Creams

Is it necessary to use a special eye cream? Is it true that there aren't any oil glands in the eye area, so that's why you need special creams?

The answer to both questions is no. There certainly are oil glands in the eye area; they just happen to be fewer and smaller than those in other areas, such as the T-zone. The only areas of the skin that do not have any oil glands are the palms of the hands and the soles of the feet.

The skin in the eye area is thinner and more delicate than in other areas of the face, so it is one of the first areas to develop fine lines and wrinkles. It may also have a tendency to be drier than other areas since it has fewer, less active oil glands. This has led the cosmetic industry to promote special eye creams. The products are generally light, non-greasy, and fragrance-free. However, you don't have to spend extra money for a separate product for this area. Your usual facial moisturizer will perform just as well as an eye cream.

Bleaching Creams to Even Out Skin Tone

How effective are creams promoted to lighten, brighten, and even out the skin tones of blacks?

The tone or coloration of black skin can naturally vary from one area to another. When black skin becomes too dry, it develops ashy tones because of the difference in light refraction off the dry, flaking skin. If black skin is injured, pigment-forming cells may be stimulated, causing spots. This is common after acne or other inflammatory skin disorders.

Products promoted to lighten and brighten black skin are usually bleaching creams that contain hydroquinone. Hydroquinone can be helpful in fading some abnormal pigmentation due to injury or disease. It can also affect normal pigmentation. However, the use of bleaching creams to lighten and brighten normal black skin may cause the skin to become more blotchy.

The best advice is to leave your skin color alone. If your skin is dry, use a regular emollient/moisturizing cream. If you have a real pigmentation problem, see a dermatologist.

Bleaching Creams for Age Spots and Melasma

How effective are bleaching creams for fading age spots, freckles, and blotchy pigmentation from pregnancy?

Bleaching creams contain a chemical called hydroquinone, which is fairly effective in fading certain types of abnormal pigmentation that is only superficial. Hydroquinone is also sometimes useful for lightening normal pigmentation.

Hydroquinone's effectiveness varies depending on the type of hyperpigmentation, as well as from one individual to another. Some people find hydroquinone products irritating; others even have allergic reactions. Most of these products can be purchased without a prescription. It would be best to consult a dermatologist for advice on treatment of your specific problem.

For information on such pigmentation problems as age spots, freckles, and the "mask of pregnancy" (melasma), see Chapter 25. Many of these problems are caused or made worse by sun exposure, so an important part of treatment may be avoiding the sun. Wearing a maximum sunblock that protects from both UVB and UVA rays whenever you must be in the sun will minimize darkening.

Topical Vitamin E

What special benefits does vitamin E provide in creams and other cosmetics?

Vitamin E has become a popular additive in various cosmetic products because of its alleged healing qualities. However, there is little or no scientific evidence to support such claims.

Vitamin E is also utilized as a preservative or an anti-oxidant (it helps to prevent breakdown of the product from exposure to oxygen). This is useful for the stability of the product but does nothing useful for the skin.

Many cosmetic companies do not use vitamin E in their products. They have some concerns about allergic reactions that have been reported. A number of years ago, a deodorant containing vitamin E had to be withdrawn because of the many reactions to the product.

There is no known reason to use a product containing vitamin E unless you like the product itself. Vitamin E is still a vitamin in search of a disease.

Homemade Products

Are homemade products just as good as expensive store-bought products?

The push by consumer advocates to use homemade products has increased over the past 20 years. Ironically, many of the safeguards against contamination, allergic reactions, and other dangers are unrecognized, circumvented, or destroyed by the amateur cosmetic chemist. The very groups advocating cosmetic safety support uncontrolled cookbook cosmetic-making. Indeed, kitchen cosmetics are more apt to cause problems than readily available commercial products.

Preservatives are needed in products to stop contamination by bacteria and fungi. The ingredients used by home manufacturers may be highly allergenic, irritating, and photosensitizing. All the recommended and monitored safety tests are overlooked. And the quality of the final mixture will usually not match that of commercial items whose formulas have been developed for acceptability and uniformity.

Natural Cosmetics

Are natural products safer or better for the skin?

Describing a product as "natural" suggests that it is pure, nonreactive, or hypoallergenic (less likely to provoke reactions). And yet, it is not necessarily any of these, because standardizing some natural materials is very difficult.

Most cosmetics contain at least some natural materials. Many commercial cosmetics use organic materials to provide special effects, making these ingredients absolutely essential to the products. Items such as lanolin, talc, powders, aloe vera, vitamins, and iron oxide are "natural," although some of them may be synthesized for use in cosmetics. Practically all fragrances are mixtures of plant and fruit extracts.

Basically, natural cosmetic products are no better and no worse than others, advertising claims notwithstanding. The best cosmetics use the best materials, whether they are natural or synthetic. The combination that produces the desired features should be used in the formulation. Select the cosmetic—natural or not—that appeals to you.

Legal Problems with Anti-Aging Creams

Did the FDA ban cosmetic creams that claim to retard or counteract aging? If so, why?

No, but the Food and Drug Administration did take action in 1987 and 1988 to require some cosmetic companies to revise and tone down the claims made for anti-aging products. In recent years such claims have become more and more exaggerated. Manufacturers say their products retard, control, or counteract aging as well as rejuvenate, repair, or renew the skin. The FDA considers products for which such claims are made to be drugs since they involve changing the structure and function of the skin. However, they're being marketed as cosmetic products (see the following question and answer for a detailed discussion of the legal difference between drugs and cosmetics as defined by the FDA).

The companies were ordered to tone down their claims or face action by the FDA for misrepresenting their products. (At the time of this writing, at least one company was contesting the FDA action, so the issue still is not settled.) It is unlikely any of these cosmetic products will be submitted to the FDA for approval as drugs; a manufacturer would have to assemble enough evidence to support claims that these products actually rejuvenate, renew, or repair the skin, or counteract aging.

Hopefully, the claims for anti-aging cosmetics will be more realistic in the future. As a consumer, you should read advertising and packaging copy carefully to determine whether the claims go no farther than promising more beautiful, vibrant, youthful skin, rather than a miraculous reversal of the aging process.

Drugs Versus Cosmetics

Please discuss the differences between drugs and cosmetics. Can't cosmetics affect the skin? What's the FDA role?

The difference between drugs and cosmetics is defined in the Federal Food and Drug and Cosmetic Act: A drug is "intended to affect the structure or any function of the body of man"; a cosmetic is "intended to be rubbed, poured, sprinkled, or sprayed on, introduced into, or otherwise applied to the human body or any part thereof for cleansing, beautifying, promoting attractiveness, or altering the appearance." The FDA is responsible for regulating the act. The determination of whether a product is a drug or a cosmetic is based on the *claims* made for the product, as well as what a product contains. Many products that a consumer assumes are drugs are really cosmetics, and vice versa.

The regulations covering drugs are much more stringent than those for cosmetics. The manufacturer of a new drug must submit evidence to support its safety and efficacy to the FDA for approval prior to marketing. Or a manufacturer can comply with an "over-the-counter drug monograph" published by the FDA to regulate categories of products whose active ingredients have already been judged safe and effective by a panel of experts convened by the FDA. In other words, the product must be safe for its intended use and do what it claims to. Accumulating the evidence for approval of a new drug can be slow and costly.

The FDA may either approve a drug for over-the-counter purchase or limit its availability by requiring a prescription. Drug regulations require that the active ingredient be listed on the label. Advertising and other forms of promotion, especially for prescription drugs, are closely regulated by the FDA. Furthermore, manufacturing facilities must meet strict standards that are closely monitored by the FDA.

In contrast, a cosmetic product does not have to have FDA approval prior to being marketed. The product's package must list the contents or net weight of the product and the name and address of the manufacturer or distributor. Also, the ingredients in cosmetic products must be listed in descending order of concentration; this is because of a fair-packaging regulation that was passed to help consumers make product selections, not because of FDA regulations. The manufacturer is supposed to carry out adequate testing to ensure that the product is safe, but the data does not have to be reviewed by the FDA before the cosmetic is marketed.

The difference between a drug and a cosmetic is illustrated by deodorants and antiperspirants. Deodorants are cosmetics because they only claim to mask or control odor. Antiperspirants are over-the-counter drugs because they claim to affect a body function: sweating.

Exfoliating Products

What are the benefits to be gained from using an exfoliating cream? Would an exfoliating sponge be better?

The surface texture of the skin can be altered in a number of different ways, one of which is by physical agents, or exfoliants. Popular exfoliants include granules incorporated into cleansers or creams, natural or synthetic sponges or pads, complexion brushes, and pumice stones. Even a washcloth can be considered a mild exfoliant.

Proponents claim that regular use of an exfoliant increases the rate of cell turnover and removes dead cells, dirt, and surface oil that may clog pores. Exfoliation is supposed to make the skin look smoother, more vibrant, healthier, and more youthful. Others are less enthusiastic, pointing out that mild exfoliation probably does not affect skin texture or appearance very much, and that the results are psychological more than physical. More effective exfoliation may cause the skin to become red and irritated, especially if too frequent or too vigorous. Individuals with dry or "sensitive" skin or skin dermatitis must be especially cautious.

Creams or cleansers with natural or synthetic granules are generally considered milder than mechanical or physical exfoliants such as sponges, but also less effective.

Exfoliation was the buzzword in skin care during the early 1980s, but it has been replaced by new fads so we don't hear much today about the special benefits of exfoliation. Maybe a lot of its former fans concluded that it really didn't cause very much improvement, or their skin was irritated by some of the products.

Eye-Makeup Removers

What is the best way to remove eye makeup?

Eye makeup, especially mascara, is generally either waterproof or -resistant, so it can be difficult to remove with soap and water. You may be left with dark circles around the eyes. A cleansing cream or eye-makeup remover will generally be more effective.

The directions for most eye-makeup removers recommend that you saturate a cotton pad or ball with the remover and then gently rub the saturated pad over the lids and lashes to remove the makeup. Most creams or gels are applied directly to the eye area then removed with a cotton ball or pad, but some are rinsed off. The face is then cleansed in the usual manner.

The eye area is very sensitive; thus, care must be taken in formulating eye-makeup removers to eliminate ingredients that may be irritating to the eyes. The products are often fragrance-free. They are often ophthalmologist-tested on individuals who wear contact lenses as well as those who do not, and are labeled as such.

You may find that a regular cleansing cream or lotion works just as well as a special eye-makeup remover. If you wear contact lenses, you will probably prefer an oil-free product because oil can stick to the lashes and get on the lenses, causing blurring and irritation.

Aging Skin

Skin Changes with Age

Just exactly what are the various changes that occur in aging skin?

When we talk about aging skin, it is important to distinguish changes that occur simply with the passage of time from those that are the consequence of sun exposure. Many of what are considered signs of aging, such as wrinkles and leathery skin with freckle-like blotches, result primarily from chronic sun exposure, not from chronological aging. Changes that *are* attributable to aging include increased dryness, decreased sweating, and changes in hair growth and facial contours.

Although aging skin is the focus of much scientific investigation, there is still a great deal we do not know about the various changes that occur as skin ages. But we do know certain facts.

As skin ages, the rate of cell production and turnover slows down and cell repair is less effective. The epidermis—the outer layer of the skin—becomes thinner, but the stratum corneum—the very outer layer of the epidermis—actually becomes thicker, developing a rough, scaly surface. It dries out and cracks, and, because increasing amounts of water are lost, the skin's barrier function is impaired.

Skin color fades somewhat as the pigment-forming cells become less active and blood content decreases, so the skin may look sallow. Some pigment cells, however, particularly in areas of sun damage, become overactive, producing blotches of hyperpigmentation (age spots). The dermis also becomes thinner and retains less water. Sun damage to the collagen and elastin fibers in the dermis results in sagging, inelastic, wrinkled skin. Loss of fat and redistribution of existing fat in the subcutaneous layer of the skin results in changes in facial contour.

Changes in nerve endings may cause the skin to be less sensitive to such sensations as pain and heat. The blood supply to the skin decreases because the blood vessels are smaller and fewer.

Hair on the face and in the ears and nose may become coarser, more bristly, and more obvious, while scalp and body hair turns white because of loss of functioning pigment cells. Various growths begin to appear as the skin ages, including seborrheic keratoses (brown warty growths), actinic keratoses (rough pink to tan scaly spots), and skin cancer.

Dry skin is a very common problem in the elderly. The sweat glands become less active, and itching is more common. Some of the itchiness is due to excessive dryness, but it sometimes persists, even when dry skin symptoms are controlled.

The skin of the elderly is more easily injured and heals more slowly after injury. The attachment surface of the dermis is smaller and flatter, so the epidermis can easily separate from the dermis. Elderly people get bruises with minimal bumping, especially on the arms and the back of their hands (sun-exposed areas). Their scars also tend to be thinner, finer, and more cosmetically acceptable.

Slow Cell Turnover

I've heard that the skin's cells turn over more slowly with aging and this contributes to aged-looking skin. Is this true? What can I do to speed up the cell turnover on my face to make it look younger?

As you grow older, the rate of cell turnover in your skin decreases. In young healthy skin, it takes about one month for a newly formed epidermal cell to reach the surface of the skin and be sloughed off. With aging, as a result of the decrease in the rate of cell turnover, the cells may stay on the skin surface for a longer period of time. It has been theorized that this can make the skin look duller and older. As the fact of the slower cell turnover time has been publicized, companies have developed cosmetic products and treatment procedures that they claim will increase cell turnover, theoretically making the skin look younger.

Dermatologists are skeptical that it is possible—or even desirable—to significantly increase cell turnover, since accelerated cell turnover is a factor in some skin disorders. Mild irritation of the skin, as from the use of exfoliating products or some moisturizers, will slightly increase cell turnover, but it is questionable whether this makes the skin look younger. However, it can temporarily make skin look better because light is more evenly reflected from the surface, with less scatter.

The Sun and Aging Skin

Is it true that overexposure to the sun is the primary cause of aging skin?

Absolutely. An American Academy of Dermatology Consensus Forum concluded that most (80% or so) of the visible changes we associate with aging of skin (the wrinkles, the leathery and rough texture, the age spots) are due to sun damage. The sun penetrates to the lower layer of the skin, where it damages the collagen and elastin so that skin loses its elasticity and firmness. Some of the pigment-forming cells at the base of the epidermis are stimulated to produce too much pigment, so spots of hyperpigmentation (age spots, "senile freckles") appear. The sun is also responsible for growths called actinic keratoses and for an increased incidence of skin cancer.

If you want to maintain a youthful appearance, you must protect your skin from the sun. Avoid suntanning. Wear a maximum sunscreen product (SPF 15 or higher), preferably one that blocks both UVB and UVA rays whenever you are out in the sun. Sunblocks are the best established "anti-aging" products currently available, and they cost a lot less than many of the cosmetic products that promise to keep skin young.

Dry Skin and Wrinkles

As I'm getting older, my skin is becoming excessively dry and wrinkles are becoming obvious. Is dry skin the cause of wrinkles?

Not really. Wrinkles are primarily caused by overexposure to the sun, as discussed in the previous answer. Overexposure to the sun also has a drying effect on the skin.

When the skin is excessively dry, fine lines may be more obvious. If you apply a moisturizer, the skin will temporarily feel and look softer and smoother as the cells are plumped up with moisture. Fine lines may temporarily appear less obvious. But don't expect your deeper wrinkles to disappear permanently as a result of using moisturizers.

Cosmetic Creams for Aging Skin

What is the best cream to purchase for aging skin? Will any of them help to slow down aging and/or remove wrinkles? Which special ingredients are most helpful?

There isn't any proof that any cosmetic cream, gel, lotion, or other product you can purchase without a prescription will reverse or retard the effects of aging. The only topical product that appears to help undo some of the changes associated with aging skin is retinoic acid (tretinoin), which must be prescribed by a physician. It is discussed in more detail elsewhere in this chapter.

The best anti-aging product you can purchase without a prescription is a maximum sunblock preparation (SPF 15 or higher) to prevent further damage, since overexposure to the sun is the primary cause of those visible changes we commonly associate with aging, such as wrinkles and "senile freckles."

While cosmetic creams cannot prevent or reverse aging, they can relieve symptoms of dry skin and thereby make the skin temporarily look and feel softer and smoother. Product selection is a matter of personal preference. For more information on cosmetic creams and ingredients, see Chapter 8.

Special Cosmetic Needs of Older Women

Can you provide some cosmetic tips to help me keep my skin looking its best? Even though I'm 75 I still want to look good.

With aging the skin becomes drier, more wrinkled, and lax. Uneven pigmentation and various skin growths may develop. Skillful use of cosmetics can help make you look your best, and when you look better you feel better and have higher self-esteem.

Don't overcleanse the skin. Wash your face once a day (at night) with a mild soap or liquid cleanser. If your skin is dry, you may prefer to use a superfatted soap. After cleansing, apply a moisturizer. Those with drier skin may need moisturizing cream rather than lotion. Select a product that feels good, is non-comedogenic, and doesn't make you break out.

During the day you may also need to use a moisturizer. Use a maximum sunblock (with an SPF of 15 or higher), preferably one that blocks both UVA and UVB rays. If you select a sunscreen with a lotion or cream base, it can serve as a moisturizer as well as a sunscreen.

Aged skin is thinner, paler, and more transparent, so makeup requirements may change. Select a light foundation makeup that is one shade lighter than your skin tone. Avoid frosted makeup. Limit the use of powder to areas that may become shiny, such as the nose. Always apply blusher to the cheeks to add color to pale skin. Avoid orange and dark red shades; select coral or pink.

Sunken temples, dark circles under the eyes, deep shadows, and scars can be made less obvious by applying a concealer cream before applying a makeup base.

Apply a lighter shade of makeup to a scrawny neck or sagging chin. On the other hand, a darker shade of makeup or skillful use of a dark contouring pencil will help disguise a sagging jaw.

Avoid bright shades of eye shadow, choosing instead soft brown, taupe, or pastels. Apply shadow only to the outer edges of heavily hooded eyes. Pencil brows with short strokes of a brown or taupe eyebrow pencil; then brush with an eyebrow brush. Avoid black, as it is too harsh on paler, lighter skin and hair. Curly eyelashes may draw attention away from puffy eyes, so you may want to use an eyelash curler before you apply mascara, which, again, should be brown or taupe rather than black.

A lip pencil, skillfully used, can fill out thin or misshapen lips. Outlining with a lip pencil before applying lipstick will also help to prevent bleeding of lipstick into the vertical furrows around the mouth (there are also cosmetic preparations you can use before applying lipstick to help minimize bleeding). Avoid harsh or dark colors in favor of bright pink and coral lipsticks.

You will find it helpful to treat yourself to a consultation with a makeup artist, who can help you select shades and demonstrate techniques to conceal and contour.

Aging Skin and Oxygen

Is it true that increasing the oxygen supply to the skin will help prevent aging?

The skin—and all other body tissues—needs good nutrition, which includes adequate oxygen. There is evidence that the amount of oxygen supplied to the skin decreases with aging. However, this does not mean that a cosmetic product can add more oxygen to the skin. Promotional claims about oxygen uptake rest on laboratory studies using living-cell models—but such studies don't prove that the final cosmetic product incorporating the tested ingredient will increase oxygen supply to the skin.

There are so many variables (size of the blood vessels, biochemical–physiological status of the tissue, and ability of the many diverse tissues to accept oxygen) that it would require a complex, sophisticated study over many years to investigate the implications of changes in oxygen uptake.

Age Spots

What causes the blotchy, freckle-like brown spots that are appearing on my face, neck, and hands? Is there any way to get rid of them?

The brown or tan spots that appear on exposed areas of skin are caused by years of sun exposure. The pigment-forming cells in these areas have become overactive. While they resemble freckles, they are larger and more irregular, and they are often darker and uneven in color. They may range in size from a quarter of an inch to over an inch. The spots are commonly referred to as age spots, or "senile freckles," as they begin to appear with aging. Physicians refer to the spots as *lentigines*.

You should protect the skin with a maximum sunblock (SPF 15 or higher) whenever you are out in the sun to help prevent the appearance of more spots. Bleaching products that contain hydroquinone may help lighten existing spots, but this approach is rarely very successful. Dermatologists can remove the spots with various surgical techniques. The topical application of retinoic acid (tretinoin), a treatment for aging skin, has also been shown to fade spots (see the discussion of tretinoin for aging skin later in this chapter, and Chapter 25 for additional information on senile freckles).

Medical Procedures for Aging Skin

Which medical procedures are helpful for correcting aging skin problems?

Among the factors that contribute to the changes in the skin that occur with aging are a decline in the level of collagen and elastic skin tissue; gravity; exposure to the sun; facial movements such as frowning, squinting, and smiling; and fat loss. Most of these changes can be partially countered with advanced medical procedures.

Drooping and sagging skin due to gravity and the decrease in collagen and elasticity can be improved with plastic surgical procedures such as facelifts. Sun damage can be ameliorated via techniques such as chemical peels, dermabrasion, and application of retinoic acid.

Bleaching preparations containing hydroquinone and dermatological surgical procedures such as electrosurgery, chemosurgery, and cryosurgery can remove senile freckles, or make them less obvious. Fibril and collagen injections may help fill in expression lines and fine wrinkles.

You will find a more detailed discussion of these procedures elsewhere in this chapter.

Collagen Injections for Wrinkles

How effective are collagen injections for removing wrinkles?

Collagen injections are widely used to smooth certain types of wrinkles, such as smile and frown lines. In this technique, purified bovine collagen is injected just beneath the skin. The number of injections will depend on the location and severity of the wrinkles. Not all types of wrinkles are helped by collagen injections. Wrinkles or lines caused by smiling and frowning (which appear around the eyes, mouth, and nose) seem to respond best to collagen injections, while deep furrows (on the forehead, for example) are helped less.

Two types of collagen are currently available. The first was approved for injections in 1981. The results with this solution will last for 4 to 12 months. The results with the newer form of collagen are said to be longer-lasting, 12 to 18 months. This form of collagen, which is injected more deeply below the dermis, is more effective for deep wrinkles. It is also used to alter facial contours.

The injection sites will look pink and bruised immediately after injection but should return to normal within several days. When collagen is first injected, small bumps appear because the wrinkled area must initially be overcorrected. In a few individuals the bumpiness persists. In others, bumps may reappear after vigorous exercise or extended sun exposure.

Not everyone is a suitable candidate for collagen injections, for instance, those with a history of immunological disorders such as lupus erythematosus and rheumatoid arthritis. Anyone interested in the treatment should first be tested for sensitivity to collagen. About 4% of those tested will be sensitive to the bovine collagen; another 1% or so will become allergic, necessitating a halt in treatment.

Fibril Injections for Wrinkles

What are fibril injections? How do they compare to collagen injections for wrinkles?

The technique and results are very similar to those of collagen injections discussed in the previous answer. Fibril foam used for injections consists primarily of the patient's own blood plasma, gelatin, and aminocaproic acid. The reported advantage of fibril over collagen is that it produces fewer allergic reactions since it contains the patient's own plasma.

Redness, burning, and swelling will occur at the injection sites for several days. The number of injections required to correct defects will depend on the size of the wrinkles or scars.

Liposuction for Aging Skin

Just exactly what can liposuction do for aging skin? Can it be used to remove unattractive fatty deposits on my face?

Liposuction has become a very popular form of cosmetic surgery in the late 1980s. It is utilized to remove excess fatty deposits and lipomas (benign fatty tumors) from the face, jowls, cheeks, neck, and other areas.

The procedure involves the suctioning of excess fat from beneath the skin. A small incision is made, then a blunt-tipped tube is inserted through the incision into the fatty layer directly under the skin. The tube is attached to a suction pump, which sucks the fat from the body.

Liposuction can be performed in a physician's office with local anesthesia. It may be used alone for cosmetic correction or in conjunction with cosmetic plastic surgery.

When liposuction is performed on the face, expert technique is very important. The incision must be carefully camouflaged, and too much fat must not be removed.

There may be tingling, numbness, and discomfort at the site of liposuction and the skin will look bruised for about two weeks. Numbness may persist for some time.

A variation of the liposuction technique called liposuction fat transfer is now being utilized but is more controversial. In this technique, fat is liposuctioned from one area of the body, such as the thighs or abdomen, and injected into the face to raise scars, smooth wrinkles, and alter contours. The fat must be carefully removed because fat that is not encased within a cell will be reabsorbed by the body and the results will thus be only temporary. Since it is the patient's own fat, the body won't reject it. The technique is still quite new, so there has been no long-term follow-up of results.

It is important to select a physician experienced in liposuction to ensure satisfactory results.

Superficial Chemosurgery for Aging Skin

Please provide information on chemosurgery for aging skin.

Superficial chemosurgery is a technique that involves the application of caustic chemicals such as phenol or trichloracetic acid to remove the epidermis (outer layer of the skin) and sometimes the upper part of the dermis (inner layer of skin). Essentially, it is a controlled second-degree chemical burn.

Superficial chemosurgery is utilized for the improvement of sun-damaged, aged, and wrinkled skin. It may be used either to peel the whole face or to treat limited areas. Wrinkles around the mouth and eyes respond especially well to chemical peeling. The vertical lines over the upper lip that cause lipstick to bleed are smoothed out. Superficial chemosurgery may also be used to remove blotchy spots of hyperpigmentation on limited areas of the face or on the hands.

The procedure is carried out with the patient awake. Within a few seconds after the acid has been applied, there is a strong burning sensation. Within a couple of minutes, the skin turns chalky white. Within about one-half to one hour, the skin turns red and swells, after which the skin turns brown and crusts form. For the first 24 to 48 hours after a phenol peel, there may be considerable discomfort and pain. Over the course of the next two weeks, the destroyed skin in the treated area sloughs off, exposing new, undamaged skin underneath. The results may last for several years. Trichloracetic acid peels, which are more superficial, are "freshening" peels. There is little or no discomfort after the procedure. Peeling lasts 7 to 10 days.

After superficial chemosurgery, the skin is very sensitive to the sun for about three months, so it is important to minimize sun exposure and wear a high-SPF sunblock whenever sun exposure is unavoidable. Otherwise, hyperpigmented spots may appear.

Fair-complexioned individuals respond better to chemical peeling than dark-skinned individuals. In some cases there may be complications (areas of darker and lighter pigmentation, development of thickened scars, and others).

To minimize the risks, it is important to select a physician experienced in superficial chemosurgery. By no means should you consider having this procedure done by someone who is not a physician.

Retinoic Acid for Aging Skin

Everyone seems to be getting a prescription for the vitamin A cream that removes wrinkles. Will it really work? What is your opinion of this treatment?

Retinoic acid or tretinoin (Retin-A®) is a derivative of vitamin A that has been used for over 15 years for the treatment of acne. More recently it has received a great deal of publicity as an anti-aging treatment, although at this writing use of the drug for this purpose had not been approved by the Food and Drug Administration.

Research is under way at a number of medical centers to determine just what potential benefits tretinoin may have in reversing certain aging changes. Researchers thus far have found that topical application of tretinoin can ameliorate some of the skin changes associated with aging, primarily photo-aging due to overexposure to the sun. There is evidence that it can make wrinkling less obvious, increase blood flow to the skin, and reduce the hyper- and hypopigmentation that is part of aging skin. Vitamin A acid produces some thickening of the epidermis (the upper layer of the skin), but it also produces thinning of the stratum corneum (the very outer layer of the epidermis). Cell turnover is increased and there is an increase in blood vessels in the dermis.

When tretinoin is applied to the skin, it initially causes redness, irritation, and peeling. The "healthy glow" associated with topical application of tretinoin may actually be a low-grade irritation, or it may result from new blood vessel formation in the dermis.

Tretinoin is not an easy medicine to use. To minimize problems, thorough instructions must be provided by a physician familiar with both the drug and the patient's particular skin. Treatment philosophies vary among physicians, some recommending more intensive regimens than others.

Increased blood flow and "glow" appear after two months, but other visible improvements—if they occur at all—will not be evident for four, five, or even six months and gradually increase during usage for at least two years.

Because retinoic acid treatment makes the stratum corneum thinner, the skin becomes more sensitive to irritation, so it is important to use gentle cleansers and nonirritating moisturizers. The skin will also be more sun-sensitive; anyone using the drug must wear a maximum sunblock (SPF 15 or higher) when likely to be exposed to the sun.

Many physicians suspect that once tretinoin therapy is initiated for aging skin, it must be continued indefinitely to maintain the results that have been achieved. This raises the question of safety for long-term use. In its more established use as an acne medication, tretinoin has been used for only a few months—or a few years, at most—since acne eventually clears.

A final judgment on the benefits and limitations of retinoic acid for aging skin must await more extensive testing and use.

Massage and Facials for Aging Skin

Will regular facial massage and facials help to tone and firm my aging skin?

Probably not. There is really no scientific evidence to support claims that these procedures will either prevent skin from aging or reverse changes that have already occurred. For example, temporarily improving circulation to the skin does nothing more than add a little color for a brief time. Of course, you may feel more relaxed and pampered after having a facial and/or a massage, and thus look better, but don't expect any lasting or beneficial effect on aging skin.

10

Shaving Advice for Men

Electric Versus Blade Shaving

Which method of shaving is preferable, using a blade or an electric shaver?

There is no good evidence that either method is preferable for all skin types. Such factors as hair and skin type, frequency of shaving, the presence of skin problems, manual dexterity, cost, and convenience influence individual preferences.

The cut hair ends are more apt to be ragged and split after shaving with an electric razor than with a blade razor. The blade razor cuts hairs closer to the surface and leaves a stubble of more uniform length, so blade shaving will produce a smoother, closer shave. However, a close shave may not always be desirable when skin problems are present.

Experiment with both methods of shaving to determine which you prefer. You may end up using both methods.

You have several different types of blade razors to choose from: the straight edge, which is used primarily by barbers since serious injury can result from improper use, and several types of safety razors. There are traditional loose, double-edge razors and single- and twin-blade injectable cartridge razors, some of which are adjustable for lighter or closer shaves. Finally, there are the disposable razors, which are quite popular today. The choice of razor is a matter of personal preference, with cost and convenience the main considerations. Most blades will provide about 10 shaves, depending on the thickness of the beard. The inexpensive disposable razors generally provide as good a shave as the expensive ones.

There are basically two types of electric shavers: the foil head and the rotary head. A foil-head razor has a thin, flexible screen over the cutting head, which moves back and forth. The rotary blade, which is less common, has spring-mounted guards over the cutters. Either type of electric shaver may have adjustable settings to regulate the closeness of the shave.

Preshave Preparations

When do I need to use a preshave preparation?

The purpose of preshave preparations is to make shaving faster, easier, and less uncomfortable and irritating. They are primarily used prior to electric shaving, although preshave preparations are also available for wet shaving.

The beard must be as dry and stiff as possible for electric shaving. Electric preshave preparations remove perspiration and oily secretions from the beard hairs so they will be dry and stiff and easily cut off by the razor's cutting edges. The product should have enough astringency to stiffen the beard, be quick-drying so there will be no moisture on the face, and have a slightly acidic pH to prevent swelling of the hairs. The preparation should provide a thin coating so the razor will glide over the skin, producing minimal irritation. Some products are more oily than astringent, acting primarily as lubricants. The preparation must not contain any ingredients that will corrode the blades or damage the plastic parts of the shaver.

If you do not have any difficulty getting your skin dry enough and the beard hairs stiff enough for electric shaving, you may not need to use a preshave preparation.

For wet shaving, beard hairs must be wet, soft, and swollen to facilitate removal and minimize irritation—the opposite of their condition for electric shaving. Preshave preparations may help enhance the effects of water and shaving cream in softening and swelling the hairs. These products usually contain soaps or snythetic detergents and lubricants. They may also contain ingredients to counteract the effects of hard water. You probably don't need a preshave preparation for wet shaving if you allow enough time for your shaving cream to soften and swell the beard hairs. Thoroughly wet the face with hot water, apply shaving cream before shaving. This should be suitable preshave preparation.

Beard Preparation Before Wet Shaving

What's the most effective way to soften the beard to make wet shaving easier?

The key to easier, more comfortable wet shaving is proper beard softening, and water is the most effective beard softener. As beard hair absorbs water and becomes thoroughly hydrated, it becomes soft and easier to cut. If the water is hot, hydration occurs more quickly, so you should wash your face with hot water and soap prior to applying a shaving preparation. The shaving cream will also help to increase hydration and keep your beard softened. After applying shaving cream, wait about two or three minutes, then apply more shaving cream if necessary before you begin shaving. It takes this long for beard hairs to become hydrated and softened.

Proper beard preparation will make shaving much easier. It seems that a common problem is not allowing enough time for the beard to soften. Get in the habit of working beard-softening time into your schedule. If you allow the two or three minutes for hydration and softening, you should find that shaving will be much easier and more comfortable.

Shaving Preparations

Please explain the differences between the various kinds of shaving preparations.

Shaving preparations include plain soap, lather creams, brushless shaving creams, and aerosol foams.

The purpose of any shaving preparation is to wet and soften the beard hairs to make shaving easier and more comfortable. If the hairs are hard, dry, and stiff, it requires more pressure to cut them and irritation is more likely to occur. A shaving preparation, then, should soften the hairs quickly and hold them erect so that they can easily be cut. A lather product should quickly produce a copious lather that does not dry out or collapse during normal shaving time. It should not cause skin or mucous membrane irritation.

Soap can be quite satisfactory for shaving, as it yields ample quantities of dense, and long-lasting lather. But soaps have to be lathered in a mug and applied with a brush to produce lather in sufficient quantity, so they are not very popular anymore.

Lather shaving creams contain soap or synthetic detergent plus humectants (moisture-attracting agents), lubricating agents, and foam stabilizers to increase their efficiency. These products are more convenient to use than soaps, but they too must be lathered in a mug and applied with a brush to produce sufficient lather. They are not very popular today.

Brushless shaving creams generally do not contain soap and do not lather. They are basically modifications of moisturizing creams (oil-in-water mixtures) to which wetting agents, humectants, and other ingredients have been added. The cream is simply applied to the face, which is then shaved in the usual manner. However, moistening and softening of the hairs takes longer than with a lather cream, so before applying a brushless cream it may be necessary to either use a preshave preparation or wash the face with soap and water. Since brushless creams leave an oily film on the skin, they may be less irritating. Individuals with dry or sensitive skin may prefer them. However, some people do not like the way their skin feels after using a brushless cream. Also, the cream clogs the razor and is difficult to remove.

Brushless shaving creams are convenient for travelers, since they don't require a brush and mug and there is no danger that the preparation will discharge into luggage as may happen with aerosol foam preparations.

Aerosol foam shaving creams and gels are by far the most popular shaving preparations. They are basically a lather cream in liquid form with propellants and other ingredients added to permit dispensing as a foam. The chief advantage of aerosol foams is their ease of application. The effects are similar to those achieved with lather creams.

Hot aerosol shaving creams were introduced several years ago but never gained much popularity. Since heat accelerates the absorption of water by beard hairs, and thus accelerates softening, a hot shaving cream should speed up the beard-softening process. However, these products cost about twice as much as regular aerosol shaving preparations and do not significantly shorten the beard-softening time. The same effects can be achieved by following the procedure discussed in the previous answer.

For men with normal skin, the choice of shaving preparations is a matter of personal preference. Information on shaving for those with oily skin is provided in the following answer.

Shaving Creams for Oily or Dry Skin

Which kind of shaving cream should be used on dry skin? On oily skin?

Brushless creams may be preferred if you have dry or sensitive skin because they are similar to moisturizers (oil in water emulsions) and will not rob the skin of its oils. They contain little or no soap and no solvents, so they do not defat the skin. Individuals with dry skin should avoid aftershave products and instead apply an emollient cream or lotion after shaving and washing the face.

Men with oily skin may prefer either a lather-type shaving cream or an aerosol foam. These preparations contain soap and/or surfactants so they remove oil better than brushless creams. It is also helpful to thoroughly wash the face after shaving if you have oily skin. You may also benefit from application of an aftershave preparation or skin bracer, as these products are drying.

Aftershave Preparations

How do aftershave lotions and skin bracers or refreshers differ?

These products are all very similar, consisting primarily of alcohol, water and scent. Their formulas vary according to intended use.

Aftershave preparations are generally applied only to the face. They feel refreshing and may soothe razor discomfort. However, it is doubtful that any of these preparations have therapeutic effects on the skin. The benefits of aftershave lotions are purely cosmetic.

A skin bracer or refresher has a higher alcohol content than an aftershave lotion and may be used either as an aftershave preparation on the face or as a body refresher after a bath or shower.

Heavy, Dark Beards

How can I deal successfully with my heavy, dark beard?

If your beard is dark solely because of heavy, dark hairs set closely together, shaving more frequently and using aftershave powder will aid in lightening the bearded area.

In other cases, the dark color may be due to excess skin pigmentation rather than to the color of the beard itself. The usual cause of this excess background pigmentation is shaving too closely, which produces irritation and pigmentation. Increased pigmentation in the beard area can also occur if you apply a fragrance product that contains a photosensitizer and then go out in the sun (see the question and answer on perfume reactions in Chapter 25).

Excess pigmentation will gradually fade if you stop irritating the skin, avoid new irritation, and minimize sun exposure. The sun will intensify the pigmentation. Whenever you must be out in the sun, always wear a sunblock. Use of a non-irritating bleaching agent will also hasten fading and prevent new pigment formation. Shaving properly (not too closely and not against the grain) is necessary to control and clear the situation. The condition is frustrating because it takes many months for the pigmentation to lighten and clear.

Problems Under Beards

I have a beard so I'm curious about what problems can occur under beards.

A wide range of skin problems may be present under beards. If the beard is thick enough, hidden beneath it may be a variety of superficial and deep infections, lice infestations, and such skin problems as psoriasis, eczema, and seborrheic dermatitis. In addition, benign and malignant tumors have been discovered beneath beards. On the other hand, a luxurious growth of hair may protect the skin from problems caused by the sun, wind, and cold. As a rule, ingrown hairs do not occur when one has a beard.

Barber's Itch

What causes barber's itch?

Barber's itch is the common label given to bacterial infections of the beard area. The infections usually follow an injury to the skin or a prior infection such as impetigo (staphylococci or streptococci). The name derives from the propagation of infection by barbers using contaminated shaving implements. However, infection may also occur if the skin is injured and the infecting organisms are on the site at the same time.

It is imperative to treat barber's itch very early and vigorously. Such treatment must include oral antibiotics and appropriate local care (proper shaving with a clean razor blade, topical antibiotics).

Pustular lesions associated with other skin diseases and fungus infections may be confused with true barber's itch.

Ingrown Beard Hairs

Please explain how shaving causes ingrown hairs and what can be done to prevent them.

Ingrown hairs are one of the most common complaints in shaving. A number of factors may play a role. If an individual has coarse, curly hair, the closely cut ends of beard hairs may have a tendency to curve back and re-enter the skin. This condition, called pseudofolliculitis, is discussed in the next question and answer. In other instances, shaving too close or against the grain can result in clipping off whiskers beneath the skin surface. Another factor is the roughness of the hair's surface where it has been cut; the rougher it is, the more likely the hair is to catch along the side of the follicle, or the skin next to the follicle, and become ingrown. Using a dull blade can result in more pressure being exerted and hair being cut on a sharp angle. A sharply angled hair seems to be more likely to become ingrown.

If you are bothered by ingrown beard hairs, you may have to experiment to find the shaving method that gives you the least trouble. Don't shave against the grain, don't shave too closely (especially in the neck area), and use a sharp blade. Shave more often but not as closely.

Consult a dermatologist if the problem is severe and persists in spite of all precautions. The dermatologist may recommend that you stop shaving altogether, at least for a while, to allow time for irritation and secondary infection to clear up. You may then be able to resume shaving with no further problems.

In extreme cases, the dermatologist may recommend electrolysis to permanently remove the ingrowing hairs (for details about electrolysis see Chapter 11).

Blacks and Ingrown Beard Hairs

I am a black man bothered by ingrown hairs from shaving. Why is this such a problem for blacks? Is there any alternative to shaving?

Ingrown hairs, or pseudofolliculitis, can be a serious problem for black men. The condition has its origin in the curved hair follicle that is much more common in blacks than in Caucasians. Shaving produces a sharply pointed hair that re-enters the skin. This causes an inflammatory response around the ingrown hair tip. Scarring can result from the inflammatory response. Shaving not only causes but also aggravates the condition. Growing a beard may offer the best solution, although in some situations this may not be acceptable.

If you prefer or are required to be clean-shaven, then you should use a chemical depilatory rather than any mechanical form of shaving. Barium sulfide depilatories such as Magic Shave® are useful. However, in many people, the use of such depilatories produces inflammation of the skin and milder thioglycolate-containing depilatories such as Nair® may have to be used. This type of depilatory has to be left on the skin for a longer period of time. It is important to follow the instructions on the package and try a test area first. After using a depilatory, you may want to apply lukewarm compresses for a few minutes, then wash thoroughly with soap and water. Most individuals can work out an every-other-day hair-removal routine with one of the available depilatories. In some cases, electrolysis of at least the most affected regions of the beard is advisable.

Warts and Shaving

I am plagued by flat warts on my face that seem to be aggravated by shaving. What do you suggest?

You should consult a dermatologist promptly. You must have the warts removed or the condition will worsen.

Warts are caused by a virus, and shaving helps spread the virus from one part of the face to another. New warts may then appear in areas that have microscopic nicks and scratches from shaving.

Weeks or months of treatment may be required to control the problem. During this period you must follow certain precautions. Always use a fresh razor blade for shaving and shave the uninvolved areas first.

Acne and Shaving

What shaving procedures are recommended when acne is present?

Any shaving procedure may be difficult and uncomfortable when you have acne. Acne lesions may be nicked, resulting in bleeding and oozing. Sore, inflamed skin may be further irritated. Whiteheads may be ruptured below the skin by the razor's pulling and pushing on the skin, aggravating the acne condition.

Avoid close shaves when you have acne. Shave as lightly as possible. You may prefer to use an adjustable razor so that you can set it on the lightest shaving position. Or you may prefer an electric shaver, which does not shave as closely and is less apt to produce nicks. Sometimes the best procedure is to alternate between blade and electric shaving. When no procedure proves satisfactory, the only recourse is to grow a beard.

11

Excess Hair—Hirsutism

Causes of Excess Facial Hair

I think I have excessive hair on my face and consider it to be a significant cosmetic problem; I look masculine. My Italian grandmother says it's normal, but I don't think so. Should I see a doctor?

Everyone has hair follicles all over their body except the palms and soles. In women, the follicles on the face, arms, and body usually produce tiny, almost invisible hairs (vellus) that are not generally noticed. However, sometimes this hair growth is so thick and/or dark that it becomes very obvious.

There are marked familial and racial differences in the degree of hairiness on the face and body. Individuals of Mediterranean and Semitic extraction are hairier than those of Nordic or Anglo-Saxon extraction. Whites are hairier than blacks, while Orientals and American Indians are the least hairy. These differences are particularly noticeable in older women; most Mediterranean women in their 80s have some degree of coarse facial hair growth. As marriage across ethnic and racial lines has become common, these characteristics have become mixed so individuals within a single family may show different degrees of normal hair growth.

Since you are of Mediterranean descent, it is likely that your facial hair growth is normal. But if you are concerned that it may be abnormal, you should consult your physician to determine whether your hair growth is indeed abnormal or excessive. Other causes of excess hair growth are discussed in the following answers.

Hormones and Excessive Hair Growth

Does excess facial hair indicate a hormonal imbalance?

It may in women. If you do not have a family tendency toward facial hairiness, and if the increase in excess hair has been relatively sudden or rapid, you may have a hormonal disorder.

Both male and female hormones are produced by both men and women. The average women produces about two-thirds as much male hormone as the average man. A woman with some malfunction or a tumor in the adrenal glands or in the ovaries may produce an excess of male hormones, and signs of masculinization may appear, such as coarse, dark hair on the face. Abnormal hair growth may also appear on the chest, lower abdomen, and extremities.

However, it's important to point out that most cases of excessive hair growth in women are not associated with any detectable internal disorder or hormonal imbalance. Many women troubled with excessive hair are entirely feminine in physique, with normal menstrual cycles and fertility. Laboratory tests, in most cases, indicate no excess of male hormones.

The cause of such excessive hair growth may be undetectable by even the most sophisticated tests, as the problem may be due to abnormalities at a cellular level. The ability to identify and correct these changes has not yet been developed.

Medications as a Cause of Excess Hair

I must take prednisone for rheumatoid arthritis. My doctor says this is the cause of excess hair that has appeared on my face. What treatment do you recommend?

Corticosteroid drugs, such as prednisone given for inflammatory disorders, for example, rheumatoid arthritis, may cause excess hair as a side effect. This is especially apt to occur with long-term use. Other drugs taken internally that may cause excess hair growth include minoxidil, cyclosporin A, and diazoxide. Excess facial hair may also appear when drugs with male hormone characteristics are given to women in sufficient doses. The dosage is all-important—in certain minor female disorders involving hormonal imbalance or deficiency, small doses of male hormone may be administered without any undesirable side effects; more serious diseases may require larger doses of male hormones with greater risk of excessive facial hair growth and other masculinizing effects, such as deepening of the voice and male-pattern hair loss on the scalp.

Excess hair growth from drugs is generally reversible once drug therapy is stopped, although this may require many months. In your case, however, since drug therapy is likely to be continued indefinitely, you should consider one of the temporary methods of hair removal discussed elsewhere in this chapter.

Excess Facial Hair After Menopause

Ever since menopause I have been bothered with increased facial hair, especially on my upper lip and chin. Is this normal? Is it permanent? Will it increase?

Hirsutism, or increased facial hair growth, is fairly common after menopause, especially in women of Mediterranean or Semitic strain. Hairs on the upper lip, the chin, and the sides of the face become darker, thicker, and coarser. The exact cause of this increased hair growth, which is not considered abnormal, is not known. The trend toward increasing hairiness may continue, although for most women it will reach a plateau, and it is unlikely to increase to the degree of a full beard.

Various methods of removing or concealing the growth are discussed elsewhere in this chapter.

Excess Hair in Children

Is excess hair in a child a cause for concern?

Children normally have a certain amount of body hair, although it usually does not become evident until puberty. The degree of hairiness is an inherited characteristic. If there is no familial tendency toward body hairiness (arms, legs, back) and the growth seems abnormal, medical consultation is advised. The appearance of hair in the secondary sexual pattern (pubic, axillary, facial) is *always* a concern in children who are definitely pre-pubertal.

When excess hair growth appears during childhood, in either girls or boys, appropriate tests for physical disease are definitely indicated. If an endocrine disorder is found and corrected by either medical or surgical treatment, the excessive hair growth usually lessens or returns to normal over a period of several months, although it may take one to two years. Occasionally, excess hair persists despite correction of the medical condition, but at least it does not continue to increase.

Removal of Excess Facial Hair

What methods are available for removing excess facial hair?

There are several different methods women may utilize to conceal or remove excess hair. It may be concealed by bleaching, or it may be temporarily removed by plucking (tweezing), clipping, waxing, or shaving, or by mechanical abrasion or a chemical depilatory. The only permanent method of removal is electrolysis. Each method has advantages and disadvantages, and the choice depends on the consistency of the hair, the area and the amount of growth, and personal preferences. A discussion of each method follows.

Shaving for Removal of Excess Facial Hair

My elderly mother has so much excess facial hair that the only practical means of removing it seems to be shaving. Will shaving have an adverse effect on the hair growth or her skin?

Shaving is the most popular method for removing underarm and leg hair, but most women consider shaving too masculine for facial hair. Surprisingly, there is no medical reason for not utilizing this method to remove facial hair. Contrary to popular belief, shaving and other methods of temporary removal do not affect the texture, color, or growth rate of hair. The hair above the skin is dead tissue and anything done to it has no effect on hair growth. Shaving *appears* to thicken individual hairs because a short hair is less flexible than a long hair and therefore feels more bristly.

In elderly women, increased growth and darkening are common. A women may clip or shave these hairs and blame the continued increase and darkening on shaving, although the changes would have occurred even if nothing had been done to the hair.

Shaving does have the distinct disadvantage that it must be repeated every day or so to avoid a bristly feeling. Also, the skin may feel irritated if a fresh blade is not used, as any man will readily tell you. Be sure the area to be shaved is wet and richly lathered. If tenderness of the skin develops after shaving, a moisturizer can make the skin feel comfortable again.

Bleaching to Conceal Excess Hair

How effective is bleaching for concealing facial hair?

Bleaching is the simplest and least expensive method for controlling excess facial hair, expecially the common "peach fuzz" variety of excess hair on the upper lip or sides of the face. Bleaching may also be combined with temporary methods of hair removal, such as clipping.

Bleaching has certain advantages over other methods because it is usually painless and harmless. The disadvantage of bleaching is that the hair is still present, although less obvious. However, repeated bleaching damages the hair, which will then tend to break off.

Commercially prepared facial hair bleaches are available in drugstores and supermarkets or a preparation can be made at home. To make your own bleaching preparation, mix one ounce of 6% hydrogen peroxide (20-volume bleaching strength) with 10–20 drops of ammonia. Either household ammonia or ammonia water as available at most drugstores can be used. If the freshly mixed bleach does not perform properly, the problem is probably old, inactive, peroxide or insufficient ammonia.

Apply the bleaching preparation immediately after mixing because peroxide action begins as soon as ammonia is added. Remove the bleach at once if burning occurs. Otherwise, leave the bleach on for 15 to 30 minutes. If your hair is not bleached enough with one application, the procedure can be repeated in a day or so.

If temporary irritation occurs, experiment with a less concentrated solution to find the preparation best suited for your skin.

If you are worried about irritation, prepare a small amount of the bleaching solution and apply it to a small test area first. If irritation occurs within 30 minutes, reduce the concentration of bleach as well as the length of time the application is left on.

Chemical Depilatories for Removal of Facial Hair

Is it safe to use a chemical depilatory to remove facial hair?

Yes, as long as you use a product formulated for use on the face. The label must state that the product is for facial use. Don't ever apply to the face a depilatory labeled for use on the legs; it is likely to be too harsh.

Chemical depilatories contain alkaline agents that break down the chemical bonds in the hair so that it breaks off at the skin surface. Skin irritation may develop after use of these products because the hair and skin are similar in composition and any compound that has a destructive effect on hair will also affect the skin to some extent. Skin irritation may be minimized by carefully following instructions and observing the time limits indicated in the instructions.

Some people believe that depilatories provide longer-lasting effects than shaving does because the hair is removed closer to the skin, but the difference, if it exists, is probably slight.

The first time you use a chemical depilatory, try it on a small area to familiarize yourself with the process and to make certain the product does not cause a skin reaction. If this happens, discontinue use of the product.

Follow the package directions carefully; the manufacturer has included them to ensure maximum safety and efficiency. Pay attention to the length of time the preparation is to be left on your skin. The time is calculated so that the hair will be destroyed with minimal damage to your skin; this varies with different products. Also, follow the manufacturer's instructions concerning the time interval to be observed between applications of the product.

Waxing for Removal of Excess Facial Hair

What are the pros and cons of waxing for removal of facial hair?

Waxing is one of the oldest methods of hair removal. It may be quite effective for removing excess hair from the upper lip and chin, but it has several drawbacks.

Waxing consists of applying a thin layer of heated, melted wax to the skin. Hairs become embedded in the wax as it cools and sets. Then the wax is stripped off the skin in the direction of hair growth, plucking out the embedded hairs. Thus, waxing might be likened to massive plucking.

Cold waxes are also available. When a cold wax is used, a strip of cloth or other material is applied over a thin layer of wax and "zipped off," removing hairs embedded in the wax and cloth.

Waxing kits are available for home use, but most waxing is done in beauty salons because the technique of application and removal requires a good deal of experience. The strip of wax must be quickly removed in one quick motion or the procedure can be painful and some hairs may not be plucked. The layer of wax must be thick enough to embed the hairs, but not so thick that it is not easily removed. Furthermore, the wax must not be too hot or it can burn or irritate the skin.

Because the hairs are plucked out below the surface, the results will last for several weeks. But you must then wait for new growth to be long enough for waxing to be repeated. This means a stubble will show for a short time and many women find this unacceptable.

Effects of Plucking/Tweezing

I have a few coarse hairs on my chin that are most easily removed by plucking with tweezers. But my girlfriend said this will make the hairs darker and coarser and increase the growth. Is this true?

There is no scientific evidence that plucking makes hairs coarser or darker or increases growth. Women commonly pluck their eyebrows without causing them to become dark, coarse, and bushy, so there should be no concern about plucking hairs elsewhere. In fact, there is some evidence that after years of plucking, hair growth decreases; the coarse pigmented hair reverts to a small, colorless vellus hair.

Plucking with tweezers is the preferred method for temporary removal of scattered hairs on the face. It is obviously impractical for growth that is extensive. Plucking may be somewhat painful, especially on sensitive areas such as the upper lip, but it has no other adverse effects.

Regrowth sufficient to require repeated plucking may occur by anywhere from 2 to 12 weeks later, depending on the density and speed of hair growth in a given area.

Abrasives for Removal of Facial Hair

How effective are abrasives such as pumice stones for removing excess hair on the face?

Abrasives such as pumice stones are among the oldest devices employed for temporary hair removal—and the least popular. Rubbing the pumice over the skin at the site of hair growth produces mechanical friction, which wears off the hairs at the surface of the skin.

Pumice stones have the advantage of being inexpensive and easy to use. They are not as likely to cause skin irritation as chemical depilatories and are easier to use than waxes. They may remove hair closer to the surface of the skin than shaving does. They have the disadvantage of being somewhat slow and tedious to use and impractical for large areas. Furthermore, if the abrasive is rubbed too vigorously, the skin will be irritated. After initial treatment, follow-up treatments may take less time since the new hairs will be short. The method must be considered temporary since it does not affect the hair roots.

An alternative to using a pumice stone is a depilatory glove. The gloves are made of a fine sandpaper shaped into the form of a mitten. The hair is removed by rubbing the sandpaper over the skin in a circular motion. It may be gentler to the skin than a pumice.

After using an abrasive, you should apply a mild emollient cream to the area to relieve any skin irritation caused by this technique.

Electrolysis for Permanent Hair Removal

What is electrolysis? How safe and effective is the procedure?

Electrolysis is the only permanent method of hair removal. It involves destruction of the hair root with an electric current. A very fine wire needle is inserted into the opening of the hair follicle and passed down the follicle until it reaches the hair papilla (root). An electric current is then sent through the needle to destroy the papilla and loosen the hair, which can then be easily removed.

True electrolysis utilizes a galvanic current that destroys the hair through a chemical reaction, but today most electrolysis instruments utilize a modified high-frequency electric current that destroys the hair by electrocoagulation. Electrocoagulation has the advantage that it requires less time than true electrolysis and therefore more hairs can be removed per session. However, with true electrolysis the incidence of regrowth after treatment is probably much lower.

The fact that instruments today utilize the modified high-frequency current has led some operators and salons to advertise that, rather than perform true electrolysis, they utilize a new technique for permanent hair removal. While they are technically correct, the basic procedure and final results are comparable regardless of the type or brand of instrument used. The safety and effectiveness of the technique depend primarily on the expertise of the operator. Many states have no standard training or licensing requirements, so unqualified persons may promote themselves as electrologists.

If you are interested in electrolysis, you should consult your dermatologist for the name of a competent operator. Physicians rarely do electrolysis themselves but may have the name of an electrologist to whom to refer patients; a few doctors' offices have a technician trained in the procedure.

Advantages and disadvantages of electrolysis are discussed in the following question and answer.

Disadvantages of Electrolysis

What are the advantages and disadvantages of electrolysis?

The one advantage of electrolysis is that it provides permanent results when properly performed. But it is by no means an ideal procedure. There are a number of disadvantages that should be carefully considered before undergoing treatment.

Electrolysis is a slow, tedious, expensive procedure because each hair must be individually destroyed. If you have extensive hair growth, two, three, or more years of weekly or twice-weekly treatments may be required to achieve acceptable results. Several months of treatment may be required to remove even limited hair growth on the upper lip or chin. Thus, electrolysis is generally not recommended for removing hair from large areas such as the arms and legs.

Many hairs require more than one treatment to achieve permanent results. Even when electrolysis is performed by a skilled operator, experts estimate that about 40–60% regrowth is normal.

There are several reasons for regrowth of some hairs. The operator is working "blindly," as the hair root is buried beneath the skin surface. Some follicles are crooked or grow at an angle, so the needle may not actually reach and destroy the hair root. In other cases hairs regrow because the operator has not used enough electric current. Since the hair is removed after treatment, it may take several weeks to determine if the hair root has indeed been permanently destroyed. (Hairs that appear right after treatment are different hairs that either were previously removed by temporary means or had not grown long enough to be visible before.)

Electrolysis treatments can be quite uncomfortable, especially on sensitive areas such as the upper lip.

Complications may occur. If the operator uses too much current, especially high-frequency current, the skin around the hair follicle may be damaged and produce scarring. Temporary complications may include irritation, infection, and spots of hyperpigmentation.

It is very important that the electrologist follow sterile procedures and not use the same needles for different patients, since there is a potential risk of transmitting hepatitis or the AIDS virus with improperly prepared needles.

See the previous discussion for information on how to locate a skilled operator.

When Is Electrolysis Practical?

What types of excessive hair growth lend themselves to removal by electrolysis?

Electrolysis is most practical for limited areas of hair growth on the upper lip, chin, or cheeks. More extensive hair growth on the face, and hair growth on the arms and legs, is best treated by one of the temporary methods discussed elsewhere in this chapter.

Individuals who have an underlying medical problem that is causing excessive hair growth may not be suitable candidates for electrolysis because more hairs will continue to appear, making treatment a never-ending process. If the underlying medical problem can be corrected, some of the excess hair may disappear and not require treatment.

It is best if moles that contain hairs are evaluated by a physician before electrolysis is performed.

Each case of excess hair must be evaluated individually to determine if electrolysis is practical. Your dermatologist can advise you as to whether electrolysis is practical for your particular problem.

Home Electrolysis Devices

How safe and effective are home electrolysis devices? Are the results comparable to those of professional electrolysis?

Home electrolysis devices generally consist of a barrel-shaped or tubular container that holds batteries for generating current through a fine wire needle that extends from the end of the barrel or a cord connected to the barrel. The wire is inserted into the follicle until it reaches the root. The electric current is then turned on, and, if all goes well, the root is destroyed.

The basic procedure with the wire-type home device is the same as for professional electrolysis, except that an amateur is performing the procedure. An inexperienced user may have more difficulty than a professional operator in determining the direction of the hair follicle, the location of the root, and the amount of electric current needed to destroy the root. Most hairs will probably require more than one treatment to achieve permanent destruction of the hair root. The procedure will therefore be quite slow and tedious.

Another type of home electrolysis device consists of tweezers through which an electric current passes. In theory, the electric current passes from the tweezers to the hair and then to its root to destroy the hair. These devices probably provide only temporary results because hair does not conduct electric current, and so the root will not be destroyed.

Self-treatment of hairs on the face may be awkward and difficult since the procedure must be performed before a mirror. In a mirror every moment is reversed; an apparent move to the right is actually a move to the left. Thus, home electrolysis devices are better utilized for removing hairs from areas such as the lower arms and legs or for scattered, minimal hair growth where direct visualization is possible.

The ultimate safety and effectiveness of home devices depend on the condition of the user's hair and skin and the skill the user can develop. If the manufacturer's directions are followed carefully, and with patience, time, and development of skill, permanent removal of some hairs may be possible.

Home electrolysis devices do have the advantage of being comparatively inexpensive.

12

The Body:
Basic Care/Problems

Prickly Heat

I am periodically bothered by prickly heat. Is there any way to prevent it? What is the best treatment?

Prickly heat (miliaria) occurs in hot, humid weather when you perspire excessively. The openings of the sweat ducts become blocked, and the sweat that cannot reach the surface breaks through the walls of the sweat ducts, creating inflammation of the skin.

Miliaria appears as pinhead-sized blisters surrounded by redness. It is often accompanied by intense itching and a prickly, burning feeling. Miliaria most often occurs in areas where skin surfaces rub together, such as the armpits and groin. It is especially common in the skin folds of plump babies and overweight adults. It can also occur on the backs of individuals who are bedridden for long periods of time.

Heat and moisture may aggravate the condition, allowing microorganisms to invade the skin and produce a secondary infection.

The only way to prevent miliaria is to avoid warm, humid environments that promote excessive sweating. The best treatment for miliaria is a cool, dry (air-conditioned) environment. Avoid activities that lead to excessive sweating. Wear light, loose-fitting clothes and limit physical activity. Take cool showers and use dusting powder afterward. A drying, calamine-type lotion may help relieve symptoms.

The condition should clear within a week. If it does not, or is severe, consult a dermatologist.

Stretch Marks

What causes stretch marks? How can they be removed?

Stretch marks occur when the skin is stretched beyond its elastic capacity. Fractures of the skin develop in the lower layer of the skin, the dermis. Stretch marks occur in many women during pregnancy but may also occur during adolescent growth spurts or periods of weight gain and loss. They may also occur in weightlifters and those who perform heavy manual labor. Genetics seems to play a role since some people develop stretch marks more easily than others.

Common sites for stretch marks are the breasts, hips, flanks, and abdomen, but they may also appear on the buttocks, groin, thighs, and upper arms.

Stretch marks usually appear as reddish-purple, slightly depressed lines in the skin. Fortunately, they will spontaneously improve in appearance as the reddish color fades. They eventually return to a normal skin color, although they do remain depressed.

There is currently no safe, effective means to either prevent or remove stretch marks. Emollient, lubricating products containing ingredients such as cocoa butter, lanolin, and vitamin E may make the skin feel more comfortable but will not have any effect on the stretch marks.

Dry Skin

I have an oily complexion but the rest of my skin, especially the legs, seems to be excessively dry. Why is this?

The oil glands on your face, and to a lesser extent on the shoulders and chest, are more plentiful and much larger than elsewhere on the body and this is reflected in greater oiliness. Thus, the skin-care regimen for your body may need to be quite different from that for your face.

Most people complain at one time or another about dry skin on the body. The condition is more common during cold winter weather when the humidity is low due to home heating, but dry skin may also occur in hot, dry areas of the country. Dry skin is a chronic, uncomfortable problem in the elderly and can lead to more severe skin problems if not adequately controlled.

Reducing the frequency of bathing, using moisturizing creams and lotions, protecting the skin from the elements, and increasing humidity can help you deal with dry skin. See further discussion on these subjects elsewhere in this chapter.

Air Conditioning and Dry Skin

Does air conditioning cause or aggravate dry skin?

It certainly seems to. Air conditioning should regulate the amount of humidity as well as the temperature, removing moisture from the air when the humidity is too high and adding moisture to the air when the humidity is too low. The air conditioning equipment in large commercial and public buildings is usually efficient in regulating both temperature and humidity. On the other hand, air conditioning in many homes and apartment buildings may not increase humidity as needed. Elderly residents of air-conditioned retirement or nursing homes may be especially vulnerable to developing excessively dry skin because their skin is already dry.

When the humidity is too low, the skin may become dry because the dry air increases the evaporative loss of moisture from the skin. In such cases a humidifier should be used to add moisture back into the air. It is also helpful to avoid long, hot baths and instead take quick showers or sponge baths with warm water. Limit the use of soap. Apply moisturizing creams and lotions on damp skin immediately after bathing to help counteract the dryness.

Flying and Dry Skin

I'm a flight attendant and frequent flying makes my skin extremely dry. What do you suggest?

Airplanes have very low humidity so excessively dry skin is a complaint not only of flight crews but also of passengers who are frequent fliers.

You can help control this excessive dryness by keeping the skin moisturized. Be liberal in your use of body lotions and creams. If your complexion is dry, wear a creamy makeup. Take along a small container of moisturizer and reapply it during the flight, especially on long flights. Be sure to reapply hand cream after washing your hands.

Ashy Tones on Dry Black Skin

What causes black skin to develop ashy gray tones?

Dry black skin has an ashy appearance due to the reflection of light on the scaling, dead cells on the surface of the skin and air beneath the scales. Keeping the skin coated with a suitable lubricating product should correct the ashy tones and relieve excessive dryness.

Very Dry Skin Versus Ichthyosis

What is the difference between abnormally dry skin and ichthyosis?

Sometimes it is very difficult to distinguish severe, abnormal dryness from mild ichthyosis. Both conditions are characterized by dry scaling and thickening of the skin.

The term *ichthyosis* refers to a group of inherited conditions that usually become evident shortly after birth. The extreme scaling and thickening of the skin has led to the common name "fish-scale disease." It may range from mild to severe, but the mild cases are more common.

The age at which they occur can help in differentiating the two conditions. As noted, ichthyosis usually becomes evident shortly after birth, although it may begin later in life in a few cases.

There is no cure for ichthyosis. However, most cases can be greatly helped with various emollients and dry-skin care. Some prescription creams and acne medications are available for more severe cases. Because of the lifelong nature of the disease and because treatment may vary depending on the type of ichthyosis, you should consult a dermatologist for diagnosis and treatment.

Simple dry skin, even when quite severe, is much easier to manage. A number of factors influence skin dryness: the frequency of cleansing, environmental heat and humidity, certain drug therapies, medical disorders, age, and the use of lubricating products. As our population ages, it will be increasingly important to understand the factors that contribute to dry skin and the appropriate treatments. If dry skin is not treated early, more severe conditions like "winter itch," dermatitis, and even ulcers such as bedsores may result.

Chapped Skin

I'm a postman, and during the winter chapped skin is a real problem, especially for my hands and face. What do you suggest?

The skin becomes chapped when the outer layer of skin (the stratum corneum) becomes dehydrated and inflexible and cracks. It most often occurs during the winter when the air is cold, dry, and windy. These conditions increase evaporative water loss from the skin, which causes the cells to become stiff, dry, and inflexible. Then the skin becomes red, rough, and dry. If the condition progresses, cracks occur, allowing substances that come in contact with the skin to penetrate and cause irritation. If the skin's natural oils have been stripped away or are deficient for other reasons, the potential for chapping is increased.

Chapping can be prevented by keeping the skin hydrated. Avoid repeated wetting followed by fast drying of the skin, as this contributes to chapping. Minimize exposure to soap and water, which can strip away the skin's natural oils. Use warm, not hot, water for skin cleansing. Be sure to thoroughly dry the skin after washing. Immediately apply an emollient cream or lotion to minimize loss of moisture from skin. Reapply as needed. If your lips are dry, protect them with a moisturizer or lip balm. Don't lick the lips. It is especially important to keep the exposed skin protected while you are outdoors delivering the mail. Carry a hand cream and a lip moisturizer to reapply as needed. You can use the hand cream on your face too.

If your skin becomes chapped in spite of precautions, intensify the skin-care procedures mentioned above. Utilize a heavier cream on the chapped areas. If the chapping doesn't improve or gets worse, you may want to consult a dermatologist.

Cellulite

What causes cellulite? What is the best way to get rid of it?

The consensus of opinion among medical experts is that "cellulite" is not a specific disorder for which there is any specific or preferred treatment.

The term *cellulite* is used to describe distinctive fatty "dimples" or "ripples" that look like the surface of a mattress. They appear on women's skin, especially the buttocks and thighs of overweight women. The fat in these areas is distributed differently in women than in men; this anatomical difference accounts for the dimpling. Examination with a microscope reveals no difference between "cellulite" fat cells and normal fat cells.

Cellulite cannot be removed by special massages, injections of enzymes or other agents, or the application of various preparations, no matter how expensive the product or procedure may be.

Hair on the Breasts

Is it normal for women to have hairs on their breasts? How do you know whether the growth is excessive or abnormal?

It is perfectly normal for women to have some scattered hairs on their breasts, especially around the nipples. These hairs, along with underarm and pubic hairs, appear at puberty in both sexes due to the influence of sex hormones. While men often develop extensive chest hair, women normally develop only a few scattered hairs. The amount of hair in either sex depends primarily on heredity.

If the hair growth on your breasts seems excessive or the number of hairs increases suddenly, you should consult a physician. Certain internal disorders, such as hormonal imbalances, ovarian cysts, or menstrual disorders, as well as certain drugs, may cause excess body hair. If there is an underlying cause, treatment may halt the increase in hair growth and the hairs already present may slowly disappear.

Clipping or careful, gentle shaving are the preferred methods for removing superfluous hair on the breasts.

Removing Leg Hair

Which method is best for removing leg hair—waxing, a depilatory, or shaving?

Any of these methods will satisfactorily remove leg hair. The following points may help you decide which you prefer (see also Chapter 11).

The waxing technique involves application of a thin layer of warm or cold wax to the skin. If warm wax is used you must wait for it to cool and set. You then quickly strip off the wax in the direction of hair growth. The hairs embedded in the wax are plucked out as the wax is removed. A variation of waxing involves applying a thin strip of cloth or other material over the wax to facilitate removal of the wax. The technique is commonly referred to as "zipping."

Since waxing plucks the hairs from below the surface, the results generally last for two to three weeks longer than simple surface removal by shaving or using a depilatory. Waxing can be painful and irritation can occur if the wax is too hot when applied. It requires practice to learn how to apply and remove the wax, so many women prefer to have waxing done by a professional.

Chemical depilatories break down the protein structure of hairs so the hairs break off at or slightly below the surface of the skin and can be wiped off. For the hair to be destroyed, the depilatory must be left on the skin for about 5 to 10 minutes, depending on the depilatory agent and the coarseness of the hair. Since hair and skin are composed of similar proteins, there may be some skin irritation. You must carefully read and follow the instructions in order to minimize irritation. It is best to test the depilatory on a small area before applying it to the whole leg. The chief drawback to chemical depilatories is their potential for producing skin irritation. The hair that regrows after use of a chemical depilatory does not feel as bristly as after shaving, and it may seem to take longer to reappear.

Shaving is by far the most popular means of removing hair from the legs. It is fast, relatively simple, and inexpensive. Blade razors are more popular than electric shavers. The chief drawback to shaving is that it must be repeated frequently if the hairs are dark and coarse.

Tips on shaving are provided in the following answer.

Tips for Shaving the Legs and Underarms

Do you have any tips on the best way to shave the legs and underarms?

These tips should make shaving easier and safer.

1. If you use an electric shaver, be sure the skin is clean and dry. Perspiration and oil on the skin can interfere with the shaver's action. You may want to use a pre-shave lotion.

2. For blade shaving, be sure the skin is wet and the hairs soaked. Hair absorbs water, causing it to swell and become stiffer, thereby making it easier to cut. Lather the skin with either soap or shaving cream to improve wetting action. Shaving dry legs can be irritating.

3. Be sure your razor is clean and the blade sharp. Dull blades make shaving uncomfortable and potentially irritating.

4. Use long, even strokes and shave against the grain so the hairs can be picked up and cut off. The pattern of hair growth varies on different areas of the legs such as the calves and thighs, so you may have to shave these areas with downward or angled strokes rather than with upward strokes.

5. Take your time and shave lightly over bony areas such as the shins and the ankles to minimize nicks and cuts. If bleeding occurs in spite of precautions, either apply pressure to the area with a piece of clean, dry cloth or tissue or use a styptic pencil.

6. It is better to shave more often and not too closely. This helps avoid irritation and ingrown hairs.

7. After shaving, wash the skin and apply moisturizer to the legs.

8. Never apply deodorant or antiperspirant to the underarms immediately after shaving. Irritation may occur. For this reason you should shave the underarms before bedtime when you won't need to apply anything to the underarm area.

Liposuction for Excess Fat

Please explain what liposuction involves and whether it can help remove fat on my abdomen. Dieting and exercising haven't helped.

Liposuction refers to a technique in which pockets of fat are removed by suction. The technique was developed in Europe in the late 1970s and has been used in this country since the early 1980s. It is designed for people who have isolated diet- and exercise-resistant fat pockets and has been utilized for removing fat from the abdomen, thighs, hips, and the face.

The physician makes a small incision in the skin and then inserts into the fatty area a thin, blunt tube called a cannula. The cannula is attached to a vacuum source, which sucks out the fat from under the skin. Several incisions and suctions may have to be performed to remove enough fat to provide significant benefits. It seems to work best when it involves removal of no more than 1,200 to 1,500 cubic centimeters of fat.

The procedure may be performed under local or general anesthesia, depending on the amount of fat to be removed. It is generally performed on an outpatient basis. The results appear to be permanent, but the procedure has been done only for a few years, so the long-term results cannot be guaranteed.

The skin may be tender and bruised for a week or more. A feeling of numbness in the treated area may persist for some time. There may be some irregularities on skin surfaces after liposuction.

Bathing Too Often

Is it true that bathing less often will help my dry skin?

Yes. When your skin is excessively dry you should wash less often and more quickly and use less soap. You should also avoid hot water. Limit tub baths to one or two per week. For daily cleansing take quick showers in warm water or just take sponge baths. Use soap only on those areas that are dirty or odorous, such as the underarms, genitals, feet, and hands.

As soon as you dry off after bathing, apply an emollient such as body oil or body lotion to retard the loss of moisture from the skin. Pay special attention to the arms and legs.

Hot Water and Dry Skin

Why should I avoid hot water for bathing and showering if I have dry skin?

Hot water cleanses more efficiently, removing natural and other oils from the skin. Thus, you should avoid hot water for bathing when you have dry skin because it will make the condition worse. Instead, use comfortably warm water. It is also a good idea to take quick showers or sponge baths rather than long, soaking baths.

Soft/Hard Water for Bathing

Are there any advantages to bathing in soft water instead of hard water?

Yes. The minerals in hard water interact with the fats in soap to produce an insoluble precipitate ("soap scum") that can leave a residue on the skin. This soap scum may cause itching and irritation.

If you live in an area with hard water, you may want to consider installing a permanent water-softening mechanism. You can also add preparations that act as water softeners directly to your bathwater. Using a detergent-based cleanser rather than soap may also be helpful since these products do not interact with the minerals in hard water to form a precipitate. These products are usually promoted as being "soapless" or as not leaving any soap residue.

Herb and Milk Baths

What special benefits do bath additives such as milk and herbs provide?

They make you and your bath smell good, they often make the bath look inviting, and they give you the feeling you are pampering yourself—but don't expect them to do anything miraculous for your skin.

Some bath additives do contain water softeners to make the bathwater feel more comfortable and leave less residue on the skin and tub after bathing. One bath additive that does have soothing benefits for the skin is collodial oatmeal. Dermatologists sometimes recommend such baths to soothe irritated and itching skin.

SKIN TISSUE SECTION

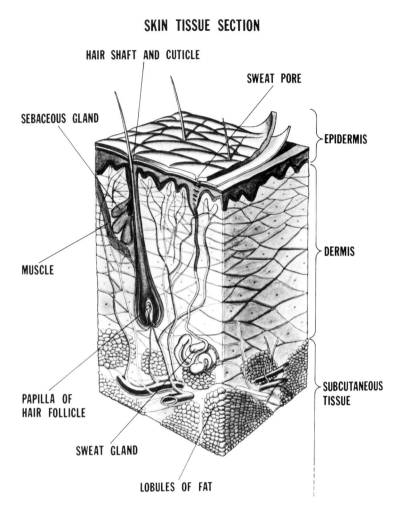

HAIR SHAFT AND CUTICLE

SWEAT PORE

SEBACEOUS GLAND

EPIDERMIS

MUSCLE

DERMIS

PAPILLA OF
HAIR FOLLICLE

SUBCUTANEOUS
TISSUE

SWEAT GLAND

LOBULES OF FAT

Children's Bubble Baths

My children love to take bubble baths, but I have heard that they are dangerous. Is this true?

Over the years there have been reports that some children's bubble-bath products cause urinary-tract irritation in small children, especially girls. The culprit in some of these products was thought to be the detergent, so the products were reformulated with mild ingredients. The Food and Drug Administration has proposed special warning labels on all children's bubble-bath products, but the situation remains unresolved.

To minimize the potential for irritation, be sure your children don't put too much of the product in the tub; measure out the correct amount yourself. And be sure that the product is thoroughly mixed with the water before letting your children get into the tub. Dermatologists suspect that part of the problem with bubble baths arises when the skin and mucous membranes come in contact with concentrated bubble-bath solutions.

The Benefits of Bath Oils

Does it really do any good to add bath oil to my bath?

Yes, but not as much as manufacturers might lead you to believe. Bath oils should be viewed as auxiliary or supplemental therapy for dry skin.

Bath oils deposit on the skin a light film of oil that helps to prevent moisture loss and thus to relieve excessively dry skin and "bath itch," a condition especially common during winter months. However, there are three drawbacks to bath oils: 1) soap and other residues may adhere to the skin along with the oil, 2) most of the oil will go down the drain with the bathwater rather than stick to the skin, and 3) some of the oil will be removed when you towel dry. If your skin is excessively dry, you will probably achieve better results by applying the oil directly to the skin right after bathing while the skin is still damp. Check the label directions to be sure that the oil can be used in this manner; some products must be rinsed off.

Don't depend on a body oil alone to adequately moisturize dry skin. You will still need to use lotions and creams to achieve optimal results.

You must also be extremely cautious to avoid slipping, sliding, or falling in bathtubs when you use bath oil because the oil can make the tub very slippery. This is especially important for older people who are less agile. Serious injury may result. If you use bath oils you should consider mounting holding bars on the bathtub walls, if you don't already have them.

Bath oils come in two forms: those that disperse throughout the water and those that float on top of the water. The performance of the two is equal. Some contain mineral oil; others contain various vegetable oils such as corn oil or sesame oil. Most also contain a fragrance, and some have surfactants added to provide foaming and/or water-softening benefits.

13

Hands and Feet: Care and Problems

Basic Foot Care

I know I neglect my feet. What do you suggest as a basic foot-care regimen to minimize problems?

Most of us neglect and abuse our feet. It's no wonder that most people suffer from one or more foot problems. We squeeze them into ill-fitting shoes and neglect to give them the most basic skin care that other areas receive. Skin care often stops at the ankles.

The most important part of basic foot care is to wear properly fitting shoes, but it appears that few people do. Various medical reports from different parts of the world indicate that many children wear shoes that are actually too small. One study showed that 48% of the young girls studied had "bad feet" by the time they were 10. Deformities of the great toes, bunions, hammertoes, corns, calluses, ingrown toenails, and nail dystrophies are among the headaches—or footaches—caused by ill-fitting shoes.

Routine foot care should certainly include daily washing unless your feet are dry and scaly for other reasons. Be sure to thoroughly dry the feet afterward, especially between the toes. Try to avoid putting on shoes right away to permit the feet to thoroughly dry. The "athlete's foot" fungus and bacteria love warm, moist areas.

While the feet have large active sweat glands, they have relatively small oil glands so dryness can be a problem. (There are no oil glands on the soles.) Daily application of a cream will help relieve excess dryness. There are also special foot preparations that provide a cooling, refreshing effect.

Once a week, at least, give the feet special attention while bathing. After the skin has been softened by the warm water, gently smooth roughened areas on the heels and soles with a pumice stone. Follow up with application of cream. Rub in and massage. Your feet will appreciate the attention. *If you have disorders of the blood vessels or loss of sensation (from neurological disease or diabetes), be careful about overtreating your feet.*

Foot powders help to prevent chafing and may absorb some perspiration. They are similar to regular talcum and body powders except that they may be heavier in texture and more absorbent. Various ingredients are often added for antiseptic and astringent effects.

Change socks daily and don't wear the same pair of shoes two days in a row. Shoes need time to dry out for a day or two before you wear them again.

Give your toenails a regular pedicure, as discussed in Chapter 14.

Consult a dermatologist first about foot problems such as warts, calluses, corns, and athlete's foot. Self-treatment may make these problems worse. Various foot problems are discussed elsewhere in this chapter.

Rough Skin on the Heels

What is the best way to remove rough skin on the heels?

Rough skin on the heels usually means calluses caused by the rubbing of shoes. They are more common in obese women who wear shoes without backs (or counters).

The easiest way to treat rough heels is to smooth them down after they have been softened by warm water during bathing. Gently scrub the roughened areas with a soft brush or gently rub them with a pumice stone (powdered volcanic glass pressed into solid, textured form). This will help remove dead skin and smooth callused spots. After bathing, massage a mild cream or ointment into the areas. Sometimes covering the anointed areas with plastic wrap or a heel cup may help even more.

If the rough calluses are extreme and persistent, consult a dermatologist.

Burning Feet

What is the cause of burning feet?

Burning of the feet may result from many different causes. In most instances, it is due to friction and sweating.

The mechanism is difficult to explain but seems to be related to the interplay of sweating–friction–shearing, as any high-school athlete can verify. Often there is also redness of the weight-bearing areas of the feet. Sometimes pitted, whitish, odoriferous, boggy calluses covering the soles may develop. It has been reported that microorganisms contribute to this situation.

Treatment involves good foot hygiene: wash feet regularly, change socks daily (switch to rougher socks or stockings, if possible, to cut down on "slippage"), alternate shoes, and be sure shoes fit because shoes that are large may allow sliding, friction, and burning. If this doesn't control the problem, other causes for burning feet should be considered. These include a variety of neurological problems, diabetes, and other diseases associated with vascular and neurological changes. Psychological reasons may be the cause or contribute to the picture.

Sweaty, Smelly Feet

What can I do about my sweaty, smelly feet?

Sweaty, smelly feet are common and distressing. They may also feel cold.

Most often this problem is due to increased nervous tension. You can also develop sweaty feet as a result of organic disorders such as hyperthyroidism and neurological disease. If you suspect an underlying medical problem, consult your family physician.

Control of excess sweating that is not related to an underlying medical problem requires a multipronged approach. It's important to diminish anxiety. Emotional support can help to reduce nervousness. Systemic medications may be necessary to reduce tensions, but they may not be helpful and may have side effects.

The feet can be treated topically with antiperspirants and antibacterials as directed by a dermatologist. Microorganisms have been found in association with the pitting and whitish maceration that occurs with hyperhidrosis (excess sweating) of feet that have thickened, callused surfaces. A mechanical method to reduce sweating by immersing the soles in water and applying electricity may help a great deal but initially it can be used only under medical supervision. This technique, known as iontophoresis, must be done with devices made especially for this treatment approach.

Good foot hygiene and care are important too. You should wear lightweight shoes with leather soles. Many people find that their sweating problems are triggered by local warmth and thick rubber or composition soles. Wear shoes that "breathe"; avoid those made of synthetic materials like plastic or vinyl. Sneakers, which are so popular for casual wear these days, often tend to increase sweating. Shoes should be aired and worn every other or third day. The insides can be sprayed with fragrance solutions to help control odors. Sometimes the cause of foot odor is found in an old, smelly shoe lining. Replace it! Wear cotton socks; heavy wool socks increase sweating. Synthetic materials such as orlon and nylon are both warming and occlusive. The feet should be washed regularly, preferably with an antibacterial soap.

The whole problem is common and has been studied a great deal because of the importance to the military and in certain areas of industry where waterproof footgear must be worn.

Corns, Calluses, and Bunions

Corns, calluses, and bunions are common problems. Exactly how do they differ, and how are they treated?

All these problems are indeed common and they are all caused, most often, by chronic friction, rubbing, and/or pressure. All are relieved by removing the cause, but they are distinctly different disorders.

A *corn* is a cone-shaped thickening of the outer, horny layer of the skin that eventually develops a very hard, tacklike central plug. The plug is very painful when pressure is applied. Corns result from chronic rubbing or pressure. They are most common on the lateral surface of the small toe where the toe rubs against a shoe. They may also occur on other toes, between toes, and on the weight-bearing area of the sole. Occasionally the weight on the stump tissue of an amputee produces corns. They also develop on the fingers of musicians and the knees of the clergy.

Improperly fitting shoes are the most common cause of corns, but they may also be associated with arthritis, feet that are off balance, improperly positioned toes, or bony spurs that push up against the skin.

Corn pads provide immediate relief by removing pressure on the corn. Numerous other products available in the drugstore will help soften corns and provide temporary relief. If these home remedies don't work and pain persists, seek professional help. A dermatologist can trim the hardened outer layers of the corn and prescribe more potent medications. Permanent relief occurs only when the pressure and rubbing are sufficiently reduced—often by wearing proper shoes or inserting special insoles. It can be difficult to eliminate pressure entirely, so corns tend to be chronic problems.

Calluses are distinctly thickened areas of skin caused by chronic friction and presssure. They may be preceded by a blister. Calluses are similar to corns but do not have the regular round shape of corns or a core. Calluses (as well as corns) are usually a defense device to protect the soft, sensitive flesh beneath them.

Common sites for calluses are the palms and soles, but they may appear on any area that is subjected to chronic friction and pressure. They are frequently found in laborers, athletes, and others who experience constant friction to an area.

On the feet, calluses typically occur over the area where the plantar fat pad is located, but they may occur on other areas of the foot where bones are prominent, especially over arthritic joints, deviated great toes, and the dorsa of hammertoes. Women often develop calluses on the back of their heels from wearing high-heeled shoes or on the bottom of the heels from wearing improper shoes.

Treatment must begin with eliminating the friction and pressure. Shoe styles may have to be changed. Wearing gloves may protect the hands. The callus itself can be thinned by soaking and then rubbing it down with pumice. In other cases keratolytic (peeling) creams or ointments are helpful.

A *bunion* is a painful inflammation of a bursa (sac) between the skin and abnormal bone. Bunions usually occur at the base of the big toe where the medial aspect rubs against the shoe. Constant external friction and pressure will thin the skin and require treatment.

The remedies are: removal of pressure by wearing better-fitting shoes, use of insoles, lubrication of the skin, application of heat, and, with more severe bunions, medical and surgical care.

Soft Corns

What is a soft corn? Are these the bumps that occur between toes?

Soft corns are usually found on the opposing surfaces of the last two toes. Usually the "kissing," or opposing, surfaces of the toes have thickened, whitish, buttonlike areas that fit together much as trains interlock. They are soft and white because of moisture. The problem is due to pressure on the lateral surface of the small toe when the toes are squeezed together. The bones in the toes provide a rigid surface against which the skin is squeezed when improper shoes are worn. Women have soft corns more commonly than men because their shoes have higher heels and narrower toes.

Soft corns are frequently misdiagnosed as athlete's foot and occasionally become infected. As with many foot problems, removal of the external pressure is imperative for relief and cure. The area can be trimmed and treated locally; placing a piece of commercially available foam rubber between the toes provides relief in most instances. In more severe cases, surgery involving the bones may be indicated.

Athlete's Foot

What causes athlete's foot? Is it true that you can catch it in gyms and other public areas where people with athelete's foot have walked?

Athlete's foot is a lay term for fungus infections of the feet. This condition is so common that up to 80% of the population of the United States may be affected at one time or another.

Fungi are molds that can infect everything from plants, foods, and animals to humans. Several different species of fungi may infect the feet. Bacterial overgrowth may also complicate and aggravate athlete's foot infections. Fungi grow best in warm, moist areas such as between toes. Warm socks and shoes such as those of athletes encourage the fungi to grow on other surfaces of the feet as well.

Classically, athlete's foot appears as a whitish, boggy area on the webs of the last two toes, with itching and occasionally pain. The area may also have a bacterial infection. The area is white because the outer layer of skin is wet. This is similar to what is observed when the hands have been in water a long time.

Another common form of athlete's foot consists of very mild inflammation accompanied by dry scaling of the entire sole of the foot in a moccasin-like pattern. Toenails are often infected in this variety of athlete's foot, with thickening and heaping-up of scaling, crumbling material under the nail. Distortion and sometimes loss of the nail may follow.

It's important to realize that many other problems of the feet—contact dermatitis, atopic dermatitis, psoriasis, etc.—may mimic athlete's foot, so if reasonable measures do not solve the problem, check with a dermatologist.

It is a popular belief that all infections are acquired from other people or from organisms shed by others. This does not appear to be the case with athlete's foot. Experimental efforts to deliberately infect healthy skin have generally failed, and a husband and wife may live together for years with only one partner infected. Treatment is discussed in the following answer.

Treatment of Athlete's Foot

What's the best treatment for athlete's foot? Does wearing white socks help?

It's important to keep the feet dry and maintain good foot hygiene. Change your socks (preferably cotton or wool) daily and alternate shoes so they dry out. If possible, don't wear shoes when at home. Wearing white socks is unnecessary.

Treatment of athlete's foot should be directed at the stage of eruption. Acutely inflamed blistering, oozing, and purulent (pus-forming) conditions are best treated with wet dressings of tap water or a weak salt solution made by adding one level teaspoon of ordinary table salt to one pint of lukewarm or cool water. Irritation by various topical agents may induce toxic or allergic reactions in widespread areas. Therefore, the judgment and management of a physician will probably be required. Oral antibiotics and oral cortisone may be required to treat the bacterial infection, which may result in elimination of the fungus organism.

Many very effective antifungal medications are currently available for clear-cut, uncomplicated fungus infections. Medications are available for surface (topical) application in the form of solutions or creams. Oral antifungal agents are also available. The oral drugs and most of the topical medications require a dermatologist's prescription, and their use should depend on his or her judgment.

Cracks Between Toes

I'm plagued with cracks (fissures) in the skin between my toes. What can be done about them?

Such fissures usually follow the accumulation of moisture (sweat or water). The outer skin layer becomes white and subject to secondary bacterial and fungal infections. The skin becomes thickened and therefore loses some of its flexibility. Movement can then result in the development of fissures. People whose feet perspire freely and who wear footgear that impedes evaporation are most likely to have this problem. Fungus infections may be present.

The area must be kept dry and good foot hygiene followed. It is best to leave shoes off as much as possible. Local treatment with an antifungal cream may heal the fissure. If not, a dermatologist should be consulted to prescribe topical and/or systemic treatment. Too frequently, fissures allow bacteria to enter and can lead to blood poisoning.

Housewife's Dermatitis

My hands have become red and irritated from household chores, and this presents a special problem because I work in a job where my hands are on display. What advice do you have to prevent this problem?

It sounds as if you have "housewife's dermatitis," a form of hand eczema that plagues many women (or men who help with household chores). While many people think this is an allergic reaction, it usually is caused by a primary irritant—that is, an eruption caused by a substance that by its very nature irritates the skin. The initial rash consists of small dry, red, scaly patches that resemble chapping.

The list of potential irritants that the hands come in contact with during normal housework and food preparation is almost endless. They range from harsh chemicals in many cleansing aids such as oven cleaners to soaps, detergents, bleaches, ammonia, polishes, window cleaners, and even food. If you are a gardening enthusiast, you may run into more irritants, such as fertilizers, sprays, and plants themselves. Pre-existing skin problems and minor abrasions, as well as bacterial and fungal infections, may also play a role.

Most housekeeping activities involve exposure to water, and water plays an important role in initiating the irritation. Repeated exposure to water alone makes the skin more susceptible to irritation by common substances that might not ordinarily affect it. Repeated wetting and drying alters the natural defenses of the outermost layers of skin, so that substances commonly encountered in household chores or hobbies can penetrate the skin more easily and cause irritation.

Avoiding or minimizing contact with water is thus fundamental to controlling housewife's dermatitis. Try to avoid wetting the hands frequently. Wear rubber gloves with cotton liners when you do wet chores. The cotton liners are important because the rubber gloves can cause the hands to perspire and become wet. Also, the rubber gloves may contain irritating materials. Try not to wear the gloves for more than 15 to 20 minutes, and whenever possible use powder on the hands or in the gloves before putting them on. Be sure to wash the cotton liners when they become soiled with perspiration.

Whenever your hands must be exposed to irritating chemicals, rinse them with lukewarm water and dry them thoroughly afterward. Then apply a good emollient hand cream.

At bedtime apply an extra heavy coating of hand cream. Wear cotton gloves or liners while sleeping to increase the moisturizing, lubricating benefits of the cream.

But the best advice is: Don't wait until you have a problem to do something about it. Take the necessary precautions beforehand. If a skin reaction does not go away, see your dermatologist.

You can obtain more information on hand eczema by writing to the American Academy of Dermatology.

Hand Eczema

What causes hand eczema? My case certainly isn't housewife's dermatitis because I'm a man.

Hand eczema is actually a general term that is applied to any dermatitis on the hands. "Housewife's eczema," "bartender's hands," "surgeon's hands," and "baker's hands" are simply examples of hand dermatitis common to various professions. This is, in fact, the most frequent form of dermatitis found in industrial workers.

The causes of hand eczema are numerous because your hands are exposed to so many different materials. Hand eczema can result from the inherent harshness of a compound or from the allergic response itself. For instance, reactions to soap are usually of an irritant nature; poison ivy, on the other hand, is an allergic response. Individuals with a history of atopy—that is, allergies such as asthma, allergic rhinitis, and childhood eczema—are more apt to develop hand eczema. These individuals may also be more susceptible to irritants or have hand eczema as part of their atopic problem.

Environmental factors in the home and workplace are also often important. These include low humidity, repeated exposure to mildly irritating chemicals, and frequent hand-washing.

Men often neglect basic hand-care practices that could minimize environmental assaults. They don't wash off irritating substances right away and don't regularly apply hand creams to counteract dryness. They also are likely to have more significant industrial contacts.

People usually try to treat hand eczema themselves, making the problem worse. Sometimes inappropriate topical preparations may slow down the healing process. Preparations containing topical anesthetics, antibiotics, and antihistamines may result in development of an allergic eruption on top of ordinary hand eczema. Secondary infection may also develop. When the patient finally arrives at the doctor's office, there may be two or three separate problems to treat. But once these are cleared, the dermatologist can usually diagnose the basic cause of hand eczema and successfully treat the problem.

If you have hand eczema that has not responded to routine skin-care practices as discussed in the previous question and answer on housewife's dermatitis, you should consult a dermatologist.

"Liver Spots" on the Hands

What can I do about the ugly "liver spots" that have appeared on the back of my hands as I've grown older?

The blotchy brown spots that commonly appear on the backs of hands (and other exposed areas) with aging are actually spots of increased pigmentation caused by years of sun exposure. Although they are often referred to as "liver spots" or "senile freckles," they have nothing to do with the liver or aging. It just takes many years of sun exposure for the spots to appear.

By the time the brown spots appear, the skin has been irreversibly damaged. You should try to minimize the appearance of more spots by protecting the hands from further sun exposure. Sunbathing and extensive exposure to the sun should be avoided. Apply a sunblock whenever you are going to be outdoors. (See Chapters 21 and 25 for more information on pigmentation problems and sun.)

Bleaching preparations containing hydroquinone may be of some benefit in reducing the color of the spots, but don't expect the spots to completely disappear. Products containing hydroquinone are discussed in more detail in Chapter 8.

The brown spots can be removed by a dermatologist, who may use chemicals or electrosurgery.

Sweaty Palms

I am embarrassed by my sweaty palms. What can be done about them?

Sweaty palms are a common problem that all of us have experienced at one time or another, but some people have continuous wetness that can be a social or occupational handicap. Cold hands are frequently an associated problem. The most common causes of sweaty palms are nervousness, anxiety, and insecurity. Thus, the problem is more acute on important occasions when you are tense and want to look your best.

There is no completely satisfactory medical treatment for all patients with sweaty palms, but the majority of people are helped to some degree with ongoing management. First, you must try to remain "cool, calm, and collected." Your dermatologist may agree to prescribe systemic medications such as sedatives or tranquilizers to reduce the level of nervousness for important occasions. In some instances, biofeedback is helpful.

Local treatment with commercially available antiperspirant preparations has limited value, but some dermatologists report satisfactory control with prescriptions of 20–30% solutions of aluminum chloride. However, if a product is too efficient, excess dryness with inflexibility, fissures, and other problems may occur. A mechanical method to reduce sweating known as iontophoresis, which involves immersing the palms in water and applying electricity, may help, but iontophoresis can initially be used only under medical supervision. Special equipment is required.

Fissures on the Palms, Soles, and Digits

Please discuss the cause and treatment of fissures that can appear on the palms, soles, fingers, or toes.

Fissures, deep cracks in the skin, appear when a thickened, inflexible area of skin splits open. This often occurs when a normally thin area of skin becomes thickened. It's comparable to what happens when a piece of wood splits under pressure that would merely bend a thinner piece of wood veneer. For example, painful fissures may develop in the thickened skin over the joints of fingers when you flex them. This usually occurs with inherited thickened skin, hyperkeratotic dry-skin diseases (psoriasis, eczema, contact dermatitis), constant local trauma, and excessively dried skin.

One must eliminate the cause if possible. Physical activities involving flexing movements of the affected areas may need to be curtailed. Fissures can become difficult to close if they have been present for a long time, during cold winter weather, and in the elderly. Active care is important in diabetics and those with neurological and vascular disease. If you have any questions, you should consult a dermatologist.

14

Nails:
Care/Problems

Nail Structure

How are nails formed? What are they made of?

Nails are part of the skin and are composed of the same tough protein (keratin) as the outer layer of the skin. The hardened (keratinized) visible part of the nail is formed by a group of specialized cells (the nail matrix) located in the white, half-moon-shaped area at the base of the nail (the lunula) and extending underneath the fold of skin at the base of the nail. The thin layer of cells that extends from the skin fold over the nail is called the cuticle. The pink color of nails is due to blood flowing through the nail bed beneath the nails. (See diagram of nail structure.) The nail plate itself is white and opaque (note the tips of the nails that extend beyond the ends of fingers or toes).

Nail growth is continuous. The fingernails grow about 1/8 inch per month; toenails grow more slowly than fingernails. Nails grow faster in warm weather, during pregnancy, and when they are recovering from an injury. Nails on your right hand grow slightly faster than those on the left hand if you are right-handed; middle fingernails grow slightly faster than the rest. Growth slows with advancing age and illness.

Any disease that affects the skin can alter the nails. The nails are

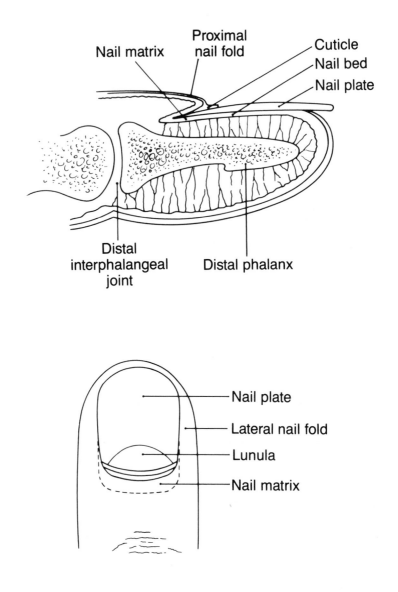

Nail matrix

Proximal nail fold

Cuticle

Nail bed

Nail plate

Distal interphalangeal joint

Distal phalanx

Nail plate

Lateral nail fold

Lunula

Nail matrix

also very sensitive to physiological alterations such as serious illness or pregnancy. In fact, the nails can help physicians diagnose internal disorders, as discussed in the following question and answer.

Nails and Skin Disorders

Is there an association between nail and skin diseases?

Certainly. Nails are a skin appendage, as are the hair and oil and sweat glands. Therefore, the nails are frequently abnormal in association with skin diseases involving adjacent areas. If the skin is dry, the nails may be dull-colored and flake and peel at the ends. The nails may also be deformed when an individual has a skin disease, such as psoriasis, eczema, or contact dermatitis involving the hand. Many systemic disorders also cause nail changes. These range from neurological diseases to problems involving blood vessels to heart-valve disease. The nails are often deformed if there is arthritic disease of adjacent joints.

Changes in the nails from disease can include increased thickness, crumbling, ridging, and separation of the nail plate from its underlying bed.

Hangnails

What's the best way to control hangnails?

Hangnails involve splits in the skin along the sides and base of the nails rather than the nails themselves. One of the most common causes is trauma, such as picking the skin and cuticle around the nail. Improper manicuring and accidental injury—a papercut, for instance—may also cause hangnails. Another common cause is excessive dryness. Dried skin loses its elasticity and tends to crack. Hangnails not only are annoying but may be painful.

To prevent hangnails, keep the hands and cuticles well moisturized. Apply moisturizer several times a day if necessary, rubbing the moisturizer into the cuticles. Avoid excessive dryness that often occurs from repeated washing and inadequate drying of hands. Wear rubber gloves with cotton liners if you must immerse your hands in water frequently.

If a hangnail develops, the tip of dry skin should be carefully cut off. Pulling off the hangnail will result in injury to the adjacent living skin.

Grooves in Nails

I've developed grooves in several of my nails that cause them to split and peel. Is this serious? What can I do to prevent such grooving?

Fingernails (and toenails) are formed by special cells (the nail matrix) grouped under the nail fold. The half-moon-shaped area that is visible in some nails (the lunula) is part of the matrix. The matrix actually extends far back under the nail fold, almost to the region of the last finger joint. Any changes in the maturation of these cells may be reflected in alterations in the appearance of the nail, including grooving and/or splitting of the nail plate. Inflammation of the cuticle or surrounding skin, for example, may be reflected in a deformity of the nail. Grooves often result from the habit of picking or rubbing the posterior nail fold, which may damage the matrix. Since the nail originates close to the last finger joint, inflammation of this joint, as may occur in arthritis, may cause grooving or other deformities. A thin transverse line called "Beau's line" may form following illness or major surgery.

Trauma, including that from improper manicuring, is a frequent cause of transverse nail grooving.

To prevent further grooving it's important to determine the cause. Has there been previous injury to the involved nails, or is inflammation present? Treatment of any underlying causes and avoiding future trauma to the nails will result in improvement in the nail structure. However, fingernails take approximately 3 to 5 months to grow, so it will take that long for improvement to be noted or completed.

White Spots on Nails

What causes white spots on my nails? My girlfriend calls them "gift spots."

Everyone has a white area at the base of the nail. This half-moon-shaped area, called the lunula, is present on all nails but may be hidden by the nail fold, particularly on the little finger. The cells in the lunula are still undergoing keratinization (hardening) and reflect white light. When the keratinization process is defective, white spots or streaks appear on the nail plate itself. These spots are very common and have many fanciful names such as "fortune spots," "lies," and "sweethearts" as well as gift spots.

The most common cause of white spots is minor trauma to the matrix. In some cases white spots occur from a fungus infection of the nails. The nail may also appear white if it is separated from its nail bed. Any disorder, therefore, that causes separation of the nail creates a white area.

Brittle Nails

What can I do about my brittle, splitting nails? Will gelatin help?

The cause of brittle nails is usually external rather than internal. They are more common in women. Nail brittleness also increases with age.

External factors that probably contribute to brittle nails are overexposure to detergents, polishes, solvents in nail-polish removers, and other drying agents.

While gelatin has been promoted for years as a cure for brittle nails, and there are even some medical reports to support such claims, evidence is not sufficient to support the value of this remedy. We are not aware of any really effective internal therapy for the ordinary types of brittle nails.

Nail-coating products that contain nylon fibers provide external thickening for the nail, thereby temporarily strengthening them. Nail polish can also act as a splint or shield to protect the nails. However, nail hardeners that contain acrylic polymers may lead to more serious problems than the brittle nails. These are discussed in more detail elsewhere in this chapter.

Nail creams and oils applied to the nails every day will help to counteract surface drying of nails but will not cure brittle nails. Hand cream massaged into the skin around the nails will do the same thing.

Nail polish should not be removed too frequently because of the damaging effects of polish remover, which usually contains acetone. It's better to patch chips in the polish. If brittle nails are persistent or severe and do not have an obvious external cause, see your dermatologist.

Infections Around the Nails

I am plagued with infections and irritation of the cuticles and skin around my nails. What can I do?

Infections involving the cuticles and folds of skin around the nails are called paronchyial infections. In acute paronchyial infections the area becomes inflamed, swollen, and painful. The cuticle may lift away from the base of the nail, and if you press on the cuticle pus may come out from beneath it. When the nail fold is affected, a pus pocket develops alongside the nail. Chronic infections produce similar but less marked symptoms. Often the skin around several nails is affected.

The tissues around the nail (paronchyial area) are very vulnerable to injury and disease. Such injuries are usually due to chemicals, water, and trauma such as pushing and clipping cuticles. Excessively dry skin is a leading cause of hangnails or torn cuticles. Dry skin loses its elasticity and tends to crack.

Bacterial and fungal diseases (primarily yeast) are also very common. Thinning of the tissue, constrictions of small blood vessels, and arthritic problems predispose to difficulty. Drying of the skin by overexposure to irritants (water, detergents, soaps, solvents, cold weather, wind) also cause problems.

Good basic care of the fingers (and hands) includes protection against irritants and overdrying. Wear rubber gloves with cotton liners while doing wet work. Protect the hands with gloves or mittens during cold weather. Lubricate the hands, especially the cuticles, with an emollient cream daily, or several times a day if necessary. Do not bite, chew, clip, or push the cuticles or periungal tissue. If you must clip cuticles it's better to clip them more often, a little at a time, than to cut too much in one session. Always use clean instruments for cuticle care. Should pain, swelling, and pus appear, start soaking the affected fingers in warm water and call your dermatologist about further treatment and evaluation.

Nail Separation

One of my nails has separated and it's very painful. What causes this? What can I do?

Nail separation may lead to infection, discomfort, and even temporary loss of the nail. Detachment of the nail plate from the nail bed most often follows trauma (a blow to the nail plate; cleaning too well under the free edge, causing injury to the adhering tissue of the nail bed; foreign body penetration under the free edge). Skin diseases (psoriasis and fungus infections, for example) and any process involving the nail bed itself can lead to nail separation. Even sun exposure in individuals taking certain photosensitizing medications can cause nail separation. Allergy to topically applied nail cosmetics and exposure to industrial, physical, and chemical trauma can also cause nail separation.

Once detachment has occurred, the nail cannot become readhered except as the new nail is formed. It is important not to clean under the nail with objects such as nailfiles or toothpicks, as this will produce further separation; instead, soak the nails in a dilute detergent solution. Accumulated debris under the nail can cause further separation; therefore it is frequently necessary to trim away the separated nail so the exposed area can be cleaned and kept dry. If there is a specific disease causing the nail separation, your dermatologist may prescribe topical or oral medications. Remember, it takes 3 to 5 or more months for a normal nail to grow out. Don't get discouraged. Covering the opened nail bed with a false nail or any other occlusive material defeats the purpose of removing the detached nail. This will delay recovery. To conceal the defect, you can cover the finger with a cotton bandage through which air can pass.

Nail Discoloration

My nails have become discolored. I think it's from my nail polish. Is this possible? Is it harmful?

Nail enamel is one of the many things that can cause nail discoloration. The discoloration is probably due to the deposition of pigment in the nail plate. The discoloration cannot be removed by polish remover. Nail hardeners and the adhesives used to apply artificial nails can also cause discoloration.

Numerous other materials that come in contact with the nails, as well as various illnesses, can also cause nail discoloration. Brown-orange nails can be caused by contact with walnuts, pecans, and other nuts, henna, iron, nicotine, and various chemicals and drugs. Nails may become yellow, gray-blue, purple, dark blue, black, or green from contact with other chemicals and drugs. The nails look pale in anemia and white in liver disease. Small, black, splinterlike spots appear under nails in several different illnesses. Yellow nails have been associated with severe internal disease, especially diseases involving the lungs and kidneys.

Nail Hardeners

Is there any danger from currently available nail hardeners? I know that the ones available several years ago caused severe problems.

Currently available nail hardeners generally contain protein, collagen, and/or nylon acetates. These products are generally considered safe unless an individual is sensitive to one of the ingredients.

Several years ago, many nail hardeners contained higher levels of formaldehyde (actually formalin) than the FDA now allows, and did indeed cause some severe reactions, ranging from inflammation to swelling to edema and subungual hemorrhages under the nails. These products are no longer generally available, although some may still be in circulation.

Reactions to "Sculptured" Acrylic Nails

Can the currently available artificial nails that are "sculptured" on the nails with a liquid and powder harm the nails?

Sculptured, molded, artificial nails are a popular means of making short, brittle nails more attractive. They are made by mixing a liquid monomer with a powder polymer and then molding this acrylic compound onto the natural nail.

When these nails first appeared several years ago, they utilized a methyl methacrylate monomer. So many reactions occurred that the Food and Drug Administration (FDA) prohibited the use of methacrylate monomers in cosmetics. Reactions included painful inflammation, infections of the cuticle and skin around the nail, as well as separation of the nail and nail discoloration. In some cases there was permanent destruction of the nails.

Current products contain ethyl methacrylate, isobutyl methacrylate, and other acrylic monomers. They do not cause as many reactions. However, physicians are still reporting reactions to these new nails, ranging from permanent loss of fingernails to marked redness, swelling, and pain of the tissue around the nails and numbness of the fingertips. The FDA received 65 consumer complaints about nail-building products between 1976 and 1986. The reactions reported included nail damage, skin reactions, infections, headaches, sneezing, nausea, and coughing. Some people are allergic to acrylics and experience various allergic reactions to sculptured nails.

Press-On Nails

Are there any dangers from press-on artificial nails?

Press-on nails are currently very popular because they are easily applied. They are either glued on with an acrylic glue or pressed onto a patch with acrylic adhesive on both sides that has been stuck on the natural nail.

The pre-formed plastic nails are made with completely cured plastic and do not cause allergic reactions. However, the "press-on" acrylic adhesive may cause reactions such as onycholysis, paronychia, and loss of the cuticle.

Press-on nails should not be worn for more than 48 hours in order to prevent nail plate damage from the occlusion. Also, the artificial nails do not always fit tightly over the natural nail, allowing space for moisture, dirt, bacteria, or fungi to invade and cause microbial infections of the natural nails.

Nail Wrapping

Is it safe to have the nails wrapped to make them longer and stronger?

Nail wrapping may be used either in conjunction with artificial nail tips to lengthen nails or alone to strengthen and repair natural nails. The wrapping may be made of paper, silk, linen, fiberglass, or more exotic materials. The wrapping is affixed to the nail(s) with acrylic glues or sealers. After drying, the edge is shaped and the nail coated with enamel. As the nails grow, the wraps move up, necessitating fill-ins every few weeks.

This technique is considered safe as long as the entire nail is not wrapped. If the whole nail is wrapped, then various problems may occur, such as splitting of nails into layers parallel to the surface, separation of the nail plate from the nail bed, and infections with bacteria and fungi. Peeling of the nails and the appearance of small white spots may continue for some time after wrapping has been stopped.

Nail Tips

Are nail tips safe?

Nail tips are artificial tips applied to the end of natural nails with acrylic glue. However, since the tips do not present a smooth surface, an acrylic solution is applied to the entire surface of the nails from the tip to the cuticle to form a smooth coating. Special care must be taken to avoid contact of the acrylic preparation with the cuticle. Thus, this procedure combines artificial nails and acrylic, sculptured nails and is potentially harmful. The same problems that occur with artificial nails and sculptured nails may occur. Also, fungus infections frequently occur after the insult to the nail.

Ingrown Toenails

Ingrown toenails are such a common problem. What causes them?

Indeed, ingrown toenails *are* very common. The problem results from the hard nail being forced into the surrounding toe tissue. This provokes a tissue reaction, as would occur with any foreign body such as a wooden splinter or an ingrown hair.

The signs of inflammation may include swelling, redness, pain, drainage (serum and/or pus), and, frequently, local bleeding. If chronic, overgrowth of granulation tissue ("proud flesh") may occur. This appears as a raised moist mass that bleeds very easily. Proud flesh causes further difficulty by increasing all the inflammatory events. Ingrown toenails are much more common in women because of their shoe styles featuring narrow toes and elevated heels.

Ingrown toenails may be prevented by making certain the side of the nail extends beyond the nail groove or tip of the toe and therefore is free of the skin. To do this, the toenails should be cut straight across, not curved as with fingernails. Wearing properly fitting shoes is also important.

Measures to reduce swelling, infection, and removal of granulation tissue should be initiated as soon as possible. Your dermatologist may be able to lift up the nail and pack cotton underneath the nail so that it is free of the toe tissue. However, it may be necessary to remove all or part of the nail. Under these conditions the nail will regrow, and your dermatologist will instruct you on proper care of the regrowing nail. Depending on the shape of the nail, it may be necessary to destroy part of the nail so that it will not regrow.

15

Perspiration and Body Odor

Causes of Body Odor

Does perspiration cause body odor? I don't seem to perspire excessively, but I sure am bothered with body odor. What's the best method for controlling this problem?

Body odor is not due to perspiration alone. Perspiration itself is essentially odorless when first secreted; odor develops from the action of bacteria on the perspiration. These bacteria are present on everyone's skin and are most active in warm, moist surroundings. For this reason, body odors are likely to develop in areas of the body from which perspiration cannot evaporate readily, such as the underarms.

Furthermore, all perspiration is not subject to action by bacteria. There are two types of sweat glands, eccrine and apocrine glands, which secrete different kinds of perspiration.

The eccrine sweat glands are widely distributed over the body surface, with greatest concentrations on the forehead, palms, and soles. Their primary function is to aid in regulating body temperature. Heat, high humidity, or nervous tension stimulates them to produce large amounts of a clear, salty sweat that cools the body as it evaporates. Eccrine sweat usually does not cause an odor problem.

Body odor is related primarily to the fluid secreted by the apocrine sweat glands, which is a milky fluid rich in organic material that can be broken down by bacteria. These glands are concentrated in the underarm area (axilla), around the nipples, and in the genital area, with the greatest activity in the axilla. The apocrine glands are closely associated with hair follicles and do not become active until puberty, as they are stimulated by the same hormones that cause hair growth in the underarms and genital area. Thus, body odor is not a problem for children and rarely for the elderly, as the secretion of these hormones gradually decreases with advancing age.

The apocrine glands respond primarily to hormonal stimulation and secondarily to emotional stimuli such as fear, sexual excitement, and pain, rather than heat. Body odor is therefore more apt to occur in times of sexual excitement or fear.

Cleanliness is the most important means of controlling body odor. If sweat isn't present, the bacteria can't make it odorous. Underarm hair can hold sweat and bacteria; therefore, removing underarm hair helps reduce body odor. Clothes may also collect odors, so it is important to wear clean clothes and discard those that have acquired persistent odors or appear to be associated with odor problems.

Deodorants and antiperspirants are helpful in controlling body odor but do not replace cleanliness. These products are discussed in more detail elsewhere in this chapter.

If these efforts prove unsuccessful and you still have body odor, you should check for other factors. These include certain metabolic and infectious diseases, some drugs, and such foods as garlic, onions, and asparagus. Discuss the problem with your dermatologist.

Excessive Perspiration

What's the best method to control excessive underarm perspiration?

There is no one solution for excessive perspiration that is suitable for everyone. Perspiration is not under voluntary control, and the degree to which an individual perspires is influenced by many factors. While heat is a primary cause, emotional and environmental factors also play a role in stimulating sweating. Excessive sweating may be related to low-grade infections, internal disorders, other medical problems, or menopause.

Antiperspirants may be helpful in controlling underarm perspiration, but don't expect these products to totally stop perspiration. The most effective products reduce perspiration by no more than about 40%; the average is about 25%. To stop perspiration completely, the sweat ducts must be blocked. While products could be formulated to achieve this result, complete blockage of the sweat ducts might produce a high incidence of skin reactions, discomfort, and other problems.

Another step in controlling underarm perspiration is to limit your physical activity. Also, provide for easier evaporation of perspiration by wearing loose, porous clothing. If possible, lower the humidity in your environment. Women can deal with excessive perspiration by wearing dress shields with waterproof linings to absorb perspiration and protect clothes from moisture. Shields are also used by men in jackets.

You should consult a dermatologist if perspiration is so severe that it is not controlled by the measures mentioned above. Among the common treatments a dermatologist may prescribe are: drugs (taken orally or applied to the skin) and surgical techniques in which an area of skin containing sweat glands is excised. The dermatologist will determine whether there is an underlying medical cause for the excessive perspiration.

Surgery for Excessive Perspiration

I've heard about surgery for excessive perspiration. What does it involve?

Surgery for excessive underarm perspiration involves the excision of the central area of the armpit, including its sweat (apocrine) glands. By experience, it has been learned that about 80% of all the sweat is generated in a very small area at the top of the axilla, and this is the area that is excised. Because the sweat glands have been removed, the area will stay relatively dry permanently.

Deodorants Versus Antiperspirants

How do deodorants differ from antiperspirants? How do you tell them apart?

Deodorants are cosmetic products that only control body odor. The package will not make any claims that they control perspiration. Deodorants may contain antiseptic ingredients but usually depend on a fragrance to mask the offending odor.

Antiperspirants, in contrast, reduce the amount of sweating and therefore affect a function of the skin—sweating. For this reason they are classified as over-the-counter drugs and include a list of active ingredients on the label. The most common antiperspirant ingredients are aluminum salts, such as aluminum chlorhydrate; nonaerosol products may contain zirconium salts. Antiperspirants generally also provide deodorant action.

If you do not sweat excessively and your primary concern is body odor, you may be satisfied with a simple deodorant, but if you also want to reduce sweating you should choose an antiperspirant.

Antiperspirants

I can't seem to find any antiperspirant that will keep me completely dry. Which one do you recommend?

None of the currently available products will completely stop perspiration flow—nor is this desirable. The secretion of sweat is an essential function of the skin, important for temperature regulation and water metabolism of the body.

The degree of perspiration control provided by different products may vary from 20 to over 40%. A product must reduce perspiration by at least 20 to 25% to be considered a true antiperspirant. Creams and roll-ons generally give greater protection than aerosol products.

Most antiperspirant preparations have deodorant properties, which may account for the public acceptance of the less effective antiperspirants. The choice of one type over another is largely a matter of personal preference for the "feel," ease of application, antiperspirant power, and odor control. For a time, aerosol products were by far the most popular forms, although they are generally less effective. However, concerns over the effects of aerosols on the environment and federal regulatory actions have changed consumer preferences. Today roll-ons and sticks are more popular than aerosols.

Deodorant Soaps

How effective are deodorant soaps in controlling body odor? Are they really necessary?

There is no question that the regular use of deodorant soaps helps to diminish normal body odor, but the question of their necessity for most individuals is another matter.

These soaps contain various antiseptic or antibacterial agents that remain on the skin after rinsing. This chemical residue then acts to reduce the bacterial population of the skin. Body odor results from the action of bacteria on the skin's secretions, primarily sweat produced by the apocrine glands.

While advertisements often indicate that we all need to use deodorant soaps, the facts are not quite so clear-cut. While it is true that these products do a better job than plain soap in reducing the skin's bacterial population, they don't totally eliminate odor; they simply diminish it, so you will probably still need to use a deodorant or antiperspirant. For most people, regular showers or baths with plain soap and water plus use of a deodorant or antiperspirant are sufficient.

Furthermore, deodorant soaps must be used regularly to achieve the best results. The antiseptic builds up on the skin with each use. After about a week of use, optimal effectiveness is achieved. One washing with another soap will remove this antiseptic layer. So if you plan to use a deodorant soap, make sure you use it all the time.

Controlling Sweaty Palms

What can I do to control excessive sweating of the palms? It's quite embarrassing.

The palms, along with the soles and the forehead, have greater concentrations of sweat glands than most other areas of the body and are common sites for localized excessive sweating (hyperhidrosis). This condition is common and occurs in normal individuals; some people simply sweat more than others, and some have sweat glands that require less stimulation to make them active. Such sweating can occur in youngsters as well as adults. Hyperhidrosis may be a real problem when it becomes severe enough to interfere with work or social life.

Emotional stress usually plays a greater role than heat stimulation in excessive sweating of the palms; thus, the problem is worse on important occasions associated with tension. At such times, try to remain as "cool, calm, and collected" as possible. Avoiding caffeine-containing beverages such as coffee, tea, and soft drinks, which are stimulants, may help.

Unfortunately, no completely effective medical treatment for this condition is available. The benefits that can be expected from any therapy are limited, and the choice of treatment depends on many factors: the degree of perspiration, responsiveness to available measures, complications such as skin disorders, allergic sensitivity to ingredients in topical treatments, or potential side effects of internal treatments.

Your dermatologist may write a prescription for a special strong antiperspirant preparation; however, these products can make the hands feel sticky and may overdry the skin. In some cases, the product can cause irritation. Sedatives or tranquilizers may be prescribed for severe cases on important occasions. Other orally administered drugs are usually reserved for patients in whom the disorder presents a significant social or occupational handicap. A procedure known as iontophoresis, which uses a low-voltage electric current, is sometimes helpful for severe cases.

On rare occasions, when there is severe, uncontrollable palmar hyperhidrosis, an operation called cervical sympathectomy might be done. This procedure is very complex and has many potential complications. It is usually done by a neurosurgeon.

Control of Vaginal Odors

What do you recommend to control vaginal odors?

A certain degree of distinctive odor is normal in the vaginal area, although Americans tend to regard all odors—even normal ones—as undesirable, because of the impact of advertising.

Good hygienic practices, which include daily washing with soap and water and wearing clean underwear, are all that most people need to combat odor. Fragrance products and removal of excess hair can also be helpful, as can wearing loose-fitting, absorbent cotton underpants. Panty hose should have a cotton crotch.

If significant vaginal discharge and/or odor is present, consult your physician to determine the cause. Treatment requires a thorough gynecological examination, both internal and external, to exclude disease, foreign bodies, and other sources for the odor. These include: small discharging cysts, infections, discharges (usually bacterial, fungal, or protozoan), and secretions from vaginal tumors. One must also exclude the presence of foreign bodies such as tampons, contraceptives, and other objects. Treatment of the medical problem or removal of the foreign object will usually decrease the odor.

Many women think that douching is necessary to control vaginal odors and keep the vaginal area clean, but most gynecologists agree that, in the absence of vaginal infections or specific medical indications, daily douching is not only unnecessary but unwise. Douching of the normal vagina can lead to injury to its lining. Strong chemicals and changes in the normal bacteria and acid medium of the vagina can injure the lining cells. Excessive douching can itself lead to the production of a discharge and unpleasant odors. Many women try to eliminate the discharge by increased douching, but only succeed in aggravating the condition.

Yellow Staining of Clothes by Perspiration

My clothes, from underclothes to blouses to dresses, are discolored with a yellow stain that I can't remove. Is this due to perspiration? What can I do to prevent the discoloration?

Staining of clothing in the underarm area can be caused by the secretion of colored sweat from the body, by discoloration of sweat after it reaches the skin surface, or by some material that comes in contact with the skin in this area.

Secretion of yellow sweat from the body is called chromhidrosis; it is extremely rare. Some drugs may also cause sweat to turn yellow. However, colored sweat is most often due to some external matter that comes in contact with the skin and either interacts with the sweat to turn it yellow or by itself stains the skin and/or clothing.

Sweat may turn yellow on interacting with a variety of organisms on the skin, either bacterial or fungal. Chemicals in cosmetics, antiperspirants, and fabrics may also interact with sweat to produce a yellowish discoloration.

To determine the cause of your problem, carefully evaluate everything that comes in contact with your underarms. Does the discoloration appear on all types of fabrics—cottons, synthetics, and permanent-press fabrics—or only on certain types of clothing? If discoloration appears on all types of fabrics, it may be due to ingredients in antiperspirants, deodorants, or cosmetic preparations (lotions and powders) applied to your underarms.

Perfumes in deodorants and antiperspirants produce a yellow staining on dress shields, slips, bras, and other clothing of some individuals. Changing to a deodorant or antiperspirant that is fragrance-free may help in these cases. Stains already present in clothing can be removed with a pre-laundry cleaning preparation.

187

To determine whether your antiperspirant is the cause of discoloration, wear a set of new, unstained underclothes and outer clothes when you start to use a new antiperspirant; if the fabrics do not become stained, you may have found the solution to your problem. If the staining continues, you will have to investigate other products that come in contact with your underarm area. You may find that using a deodorant instead of an antiperspirant solves the problem.

If all these efforts fail, you may want to consult a dermatologist to determine whether your condition is due to bacterial or fungal infection, drugs, or other medical problems; control of the underlying cause will control the yellow staining.

Prickly Heat

What causes prickly heat? What treatment is advised?

Prickly heat (miliaria) is caused by temporary blockage of the sweat duct openings on the skin surface. When sweat cannot reach the skin's surface and a person is subjected to a stimulus that provokes sweating, the newly formed sweat may break through the wall of the sweat duct and create an inflammatory response in the skin. The lesions of prickly heat appear as pinhead-sized clear blisters. The lesions are usually accompanied by itching and burning. Heat and moisture may aggravate the condition and allow microorganisms to invade, producing a secondary infection.

Miliaria is especially common in areas which skin surfaces are close together. Thus, it commonly occurs in the skin folds of plump babies and overweight adults.

An important part of treatment is keeping the skin cool and dry. Light, loose-fitting clothes, air conditioning or fans, cool showers followed by the use of dusting powder, and limiting physical activity are helpful. Babies with prickly heat should be gently bathed in plain water, or water plus a mild soap. A physician should be consulted if the prickly heat is severe or does not respond to therapy.

16

Allergy and Irritation

Allergy Versus Irritation

What is the difference between skin allergies and skin irritation?

The term *allergy* refers to an altered reaction (allergy) to a specific material (allergen). Allergy involves the immune system. A specific allergy may be either rare or common—but even the common ones will never affect 100% of those exposed to that allergen.

Skin *irritation* is caused by a material that can cause a reaction in 100% of those in contact with the irritant under the appropriate circumstances. There is no altered reactivity in irritant responses and they do not involve the immune system. Other factors are the nature of the skin surface (palms versus backs of hands), length of contact, subject's age, occlusion, and concentration of material.

A chemical can be both an allergen (cause an allergic response) and an irritant (cause an irritative response). Frequently, the resulting rashes can be distinguished by their appearance,which may be very different. However, sometimes the rashes are indistinguishable in spite of the different mechanisms involved. A commonly used item that most often produces an irritative response, but may sometimes produce an allergic one, is soap. Ordinarily, one application of soap does not provoke a reaction to its irritant qualities because it is diluted with water and rinsed off. However, with repeated washings, soap may cause irritation. If soap shavings are applied to the skin, covered, and left in place for 24 to 48 hours, irritation of the skin will follow. In contrast, the chemical contained in the poison ivy plant (urishiol) is rarely an irritant, but it is a common allergen, producing allergic contact dermatitis. An irritant material may be shown to be an allergen only after it is diluted below its irritance level. In fact, the materials used to test for allergic contact dermatitis must be diluted to the extent that they do not cause irrative responses.

Individuals who suspect that they are allergic to a chemical or product can apply it to a small area of the skin, such as inside the elbow, for several days to determine if they are sensitive to the material, but this in itself does not rule out the potential for a reaction if the substance is applied to other areas in the future.

Hives

Exactly what are hives? What causes them?

Hives (urticaria) are localized swellings (wheals) of the skin or mucous membranes that usually occur in groups. They can appear on any area of the skin. They usually last about 1 to 6 hours before fading away, leaving no trace. No single hive lasts more than 36 hours. But bouts of urticaria can be chronic, occurring almost daily and lasting 3 to 6 weeks. About 20% of the population will have hives sometime during their lives.

Hives vary in size from as small as a pencil eraser to as large as a dinner plate, and may join together to form larger hives. When they are forming, the swollen area may itch, burn, or sting.

While the cause of hives is usually not evident, the possibilities include medications, foods, inhalants, infections, and infestations. Some materials may cause wheals after contacting the skin; this condition is known as contact urticaria. Some cases of hives may be related to emotional stress. A special type of hives may result from rapid changes in temperature. These hives are distinctive. They appear as small, puffy lesions surrounded by large, flat, red areas. Certain people can develop hives from sunlight or cold temperatures. Dermographism is a form of hives elicited by physical pressure, for example, by snugly fitting elasticized garments.

The best treatment for hives is to determine the cause and then eliminate it. However, finding the cause of hives requires good observation and historical information. A careful history taken by a dermatologist and appropriate tests, if indicated, may successfully identify the causative factors. However, in a significant number of cases, the cause of hives is never identified.

Medications such as antihistamines and systemic corticosteroids will help to control urticaria. Topical remedies offer symptomatic relief. For more details about hives, write to the American Academy of Dermatology.

Reactions to Jewelry and Other Metals

What causes me to break out in a rash when I wear costume jewelry? Even my watch causes a reaction.

The culprit is probably nickel, which is present in many metal objects, including the backs of watch cases and bands, costume jewelry, zippers, hairpins, eyelash curlers, hair curlers, purse clasps, thimbles, needles, scissors, coins, hooks on bras, belt buckles, metal buttons on jeans, eyeglass frames, identification tags ... the list is endless. It's estimated that about 10% of the population is allergic to nickel, with more women than men (20 to 1) affected because women wear more jewelry than men.

Nickel is used in various alloys and thus has many disguises. These alloys include white gold, German silver, and such strange-sounding metals as Alnico, Ticonium, and Invar. Also, many so-called chrome-plated objects contain enough nickel to produce a reaction in nickel-sensitive people.

Sweating greatly increases the degree of dermatitis in nickel-sensitive people. In the summertime, when people perspire freely, a woman sensitive to nickel may find that costume jewelry or clothing accessories will cause an itchy, prickly sensation within 15 to 20 minutes after contact with the skin; a rash may appear within an hour. When not perspiring, the same woman might be able to wear nickel-plated objects for several hours without showing any symptoms.

The diagnosis of nickel dermatitis is simple because it occurs on the area of skin in contact with the metal. A rash will occur on the earlobes where earrings have been in touch with the skin; if a watch is to blame the rash will occur on the wrist underneath the back and/or band. If you eliminate contact with the offending object, the rash will generally disappear within a few days. For more severe reactions your dermatologist can prescribe a corticosteroid cream.

Your dermatologist can perform a patch test to confirm

whether you are indeed allergic to nickel. If you are allergic, you should try to avoid contact with metals that contain nickel.

Coating jewelry with clear lacquer or nail polish may help minimize reactions. Sterling silver and 18-karat gold may contain nickel. Many nickel-allergic people can also tolerate stainless steel.

Reactions to Preservatives in Products

I understand that preservatives may cause allergic reactions to cosmetics. If this is so, why are they used? Which preservatives should I be wary of?

Preservatives are added to products to protect them from spoilage or contamination during use; thus, they are important ingredients. Unfortunately, they sometimes produce allergic reactions, although the incidence is low.

Skin reactions to preservatives in cosmetics and topical medications usually appear as dermatitis (or eczema) with redness, scaling, swelling, blisters, oozing, or cracking of the skin. The reaction may be mild or severe and is usually associated with burning or itching. Such reactions may appear as hives or occasionally as just local swelling. More commonly, a reaction may occur, often for the first time, when products are used on damaged or irritated skin. Ingestion of some preservatives in foods or medications will produce skin reactions and may induce sensitization.

The most common preservatives named as potential sensitizers are formalin, formalin-releasing compounds, parabens, and methylchloro- and methylisothiazolinone. Yet other preservatives, including sorbic acid, vitamin E, and vitamin C, have also caused allergic reactions. Some are implicated more than others either because they have a greater potential to produce reactions or because the particular preservative may be used more commonly in cosmetics and topical medications as well as floor wax, shoe polish, cutting oils, and other products. A preservative is chosen on the basis of its efficiency, cost, and stability, and whether it can be used in a particular mixture.

Because preservatives are present in so many diverse products used at home and in the workplace, it is difficult to avoid them. Patch and use testing are the best methods to substantiate the diagnosis of allergic contact dermatitis to preservatives.

If you are sensitive to a particular preservative, you should check the ingredient listing on a cosmetic product before purchasing it. All cosmetic products must list ingredients on the outer carton. Preservatives are listed near the end because ingredients are listed in descending order of concentration and the concentration of preservatives is very low.

Reactions to Soaps and Detergents

Are allergic reactions to soaps and detergents common? What about irritation?

Allergy to soaps and detergents per se is not very common, but allergic reactions to the fragrance, color, or antibacterial ingredients in the products may occur. Irritant reactions to soap and detergents are far more common than allergic reactions. The scientific or biological reasons for irritation are not entirely understood, but damage to the skin's barrier (stratum corneum) leads to damage of the epidermis and inflammation. Itching and burning are the usual signals that the skin has become damaged.

Fortunately, soap is diluted with water during use and then rinsed off the skin. This leaves little or no residue on the skin, so the chances for irritation are reduced. To avoid irritant reactions, minimize overdrying the skin by too frequent washing. Application of an oily lotion, a cream, or an oil will be protective and prevent difficulties. Wearing rubber gloves when working with water, soaps, and solvents will add additional protection.

If an allergic reaction is suspected, consult a dermatologist.

Allergy to Shoe Leather

What causes allergic reactions to shoe leather?

Shoe leather is treated, dyed, and preserved with many chemicals so it will be durable, flexible, and mildew-proof. Allergic reactions to shoe leather may be due to such chemicals as well as dyes, antimicrobial and antifungal compounds, chromates, rubber, glues, antioxidants, and other substances used in the manufacture and treatment of the leather. Stockings and socks put a partial barrier between the skin and inner surface of the shoe. Reactions to shoes are more common in those whose feet perspire profusely and in hot, humid environments. Shoes should be allowed to dry completely before they are worn again.

While sandals will promote dryness of the feet, they may present problems because they are more likely to be worn without socks. Sandals (and other shoes) made in foreign countries may cause special problems; for example, sandals from the Indian subcontinent are treated with a chemical related to poison ivy, so a person sensitive to poison ivy will develop poison ivy dermatitis from wearing these sandals.

If one suspects an allergic reaction, patch testing and use tests should be performed under the supervision of a dermatologist. Conditions that may be confused with contact dermatitis of the feet from shoe leather include eczema, fungus infections, and psoriasis. Treatment requires proper diagnosis and expert management, which often must be individualized. Topical corticosteroid preparations are the mainstay of any treatment regimen.

Allergies to Wool

Are some people allergic to wool?

Yes, people can definitely be allergic to wool. Such allergic reactions may be due to materials adhering to the wool, the wool itself, or wool dust (which can be inhaled). But many so-called "allergic reactions" to wool are secondary to contact with the rough prickly surface of woolen materials. Some wool has a minute amount of lanolin on its fibers; this residual lanolin, as well as dyes and other chemicals, may be the allergens rather than pure, absolutely clean wool fibers.

Allergies to Lanolin

Are people really allergic to lanolin?

Yes. Allergic reactions to lanolin are common. Some investigators believe that as much as 5% of the population is allergic to lanolin; others believe the incidence is lower.

Lanolin is a valuable ingredient in many products, including cosmetics, furniture and shoe polish, floor and car waxes, and dozens of other products. Thus, much research by industry has been devoted to identifying and eliminating the offending fractions responsible for allergic reactions from lanolin. Today, these modified lanolin derivatives, which have less potential to produce allergic reactions, are most often used in products that come in contact with the skin.

Reactions to Stretch Garments

I break out in a rash whenever I wear stretch fabric bras or other undergarments. What causes this reaction?

You may be allergic to the rubber or spandex that gives the fabric its stretchability. Rubber products frequently cause allergic contact dermatitis.

Rubber is found in innumerable products in one form or another. Natural rubber alone is practically never a sensitizer. Rather, it is the various chemicals that are added to the rubber to preserve it and improve its quality that cause allergic contact dermatitis. People who are sensitive to rubber products must look for substitutes.

Many stretchable garments are now being made of spandex, a synthetic elastic fiber. Spandex is used in various foundation garments, swimsuits, surgical bandages, and support hose. When first introduced, some spandex fibers contained additives that were sensitizers, but these additives have been removed from currently available spandex. Today, spandex rarely, if ever, produces allergic reactions.

Individuals who are sensitive to rubber can wear foundation garments made of spandex if the garments do not have rubber-backed fasteners or edges. Certain manufacturers produce girdles and brassieres that are completely rubber-free.

Elasticized clothing may also cause skin reactions as a consequence of mechanical pressure (fitting too snugly). These reactions include hives, acnelike blemishes, and redness. Pre-existing dermatoses may be aggravated.

Your dermatologist can help provide information on the cause of your particular reaction.

Allergic Reactions to Hair Dyes

If I am allergic to permanent hair dyes will I react to other hair dyes or dyes used in fabrics?

You may. While thousands and thousands of people color their hair without experiencing a reaction, a few will become allergic to paraphenylenediamine (PPD), the dye utilized in permanent tints. Once a person is sensitized to PPD, he or she may also become allergic to substances that are its close chemical relatives, including other types of dyes used to color hair or clothing as well as certain medications, through a process known as cross-sensitization.

If you are allergic to PPD you may also react to the aniline dyes used in semi-permanent hair coloring products and even temporary coloring products that contain azo dyes, so you should do a patch test before using any of these products. Alternatives include the use of vegetable (henna) dye or metallic salt dyes, both of which have certain drawbacks. For a detailed discussion of the various types of hair dyes, see Chapter 4.

PPD dyes are rarely used in any clothing except furs. The azo and aniline dyes, however, are used in wearing apparel and, since they may produce cross-reactions with PPD, individuals sensitive to PPD may not be able to wear dark clothes (black, blue, brown, and dark gray). They often have no difficulty wearing fabrics that have been dyed in lighter shades.

Certain widely used local anesthetics such as procaine and benzocaine are chemical relatives of PPD compounds. About one-fourth of people with PPD sensitivity are also allergic to these anesthetics; therefore, you should tell your doctor or dentist about your allergic reaction to PPD before you are given any local anesthetic. Lidocaine (Xylocaine®) and mepivacaine (Carbocaine®) are local anesthetics that may be substituted for procaine and benzocaine.

The chemical sunscreen para-aminobenzoic acid (PABA) and its salts, which are the active ingredients in many sunscreen products, may also cross-react with PPD. In such cases, an individual must use a PABA-free product. Several PABA-free sunscreens are now available.

Your dermatologist can help you determine whether you will cross-react to these other dyes and related chemicals via patch testing.

Poison Ivy Dermatitis

Please provide information on what to do about poison ivy. How does the reaction spread?

The poison ivy (rhus) plant family includes poison ivy, poison oak, and poison sumac. One or more of the plants is found in every state in the continental United States. The oily resin (oleoresin) found on all parts of the plants contains compounds called catechols, which are potent allergens capable of causing skin eruptions in many people who come in contact with the plants.

All the rhus plants produce an identical dermatitis, the symptoms of which are reddening of the skin and blistering, almost always accompanied by itching. The extent of the dermatitis depends on the skin areas with which the plant has been in contact, and the severity of the eruption depends on both the amount of plant material deposited at a particular site and the degree of allergic sensitivity of the individual. The more allergic a person is to poison ivy plants and the more of the plant material left on the skin, the more intense the reaction.

Poison ivy does not really "spread." The skin reaction appears to spread because the time required for the lesions to appear depends on the amount of oleoresin deposited on the skin. Areas that have more oleoresin will develop a reaction quicker and will be more severely involved than areas that had less contact with the oleoresin. The lesions often appear in straight lines because the victim has brushed against the plant.

If you come in contact with poison ivy or one of the other plants in the rhus family, it is important that you remove the oleoresin from the skin with soap and water as soon as possible. If this is done within 30 minutes you are likely to prevent the development of poison ivy dermatitis, or at least reduce its severity significantly. It is very important to thoroughly wash the hands, including the skin under the fingernails, because if contaminated, they can spread the allergen to other areas of your body. Also, wash all clothes, gloves, garden implements—anything that may have come in contact with the plant.

The application of cold water compresses to the affected areas will provide relief from itching and reduce the inflammation. Contrary to popular superstition, bathing, showering, and other exposures to water are useful, not detrimental. Calamine lotion, applied early, will hasten the drying of small blisters. Extensive eruptions may be treated by physicians with local or systemic corticosteroids, and superimposed infections are treated with antibiotics. Antihistamine drugs given orally often relieve the itching.

The best way to prevent poison ivy dermatitis is to avoid the plants that cause it. Follow the old adage "leaflets three, let it be." On all the rhus plants except poison sumac, each leaf comprises three leaflets that arise from a node on the stem. The leaves, therefore, are never seen in pairs. The leaf of poison sumac con-

197

sists of 7 to 13 paired leaflets (plus the sole terminal leaflet) along a straight midrib.

If you become allergic to our native poison ivy plants, you will often become allergic to several plant oils derived from other countries. A furniture lacquer obtained from the Japanese lacquer tree contains such an oil. So does the rind of a mango and the shell of the cashew nut. Voodoo dolls imported from Haiti and stirring sticks made from cashew nuts may produce a poison-ivy-like dermatitis.

You can obtain more information on poison plant reactions from the American Academy of Dermatology.

Atopic Dermatitis

Atopic dermatitis sounds like such a strange disease, but I understand that it is just an allergy. Please provide more details.

The term "atopy" literally means "without place." The term was coined to describe a strange disease. The adjective "atopic" designates a group of allergic or associated diseases that often occur in several members of the same family. Many members of these families suffer not only from allergies such as hay fever and asthma but also from skin eruptions called atopic dermatitis. It affects about 3–5% of the population.

The disease occurs at all ages but mainly from infancy to young adulthood. The lesions are excruciatingly itchy. When the disease starts in infancy, it is called infantile eczema. Infantile eczema is characterized by an itching, oozing, crusting dermatitis that tends to be localized principally on the face and scalp, although spots can appear at other sites. If the disease continues or recurs beyond infancy, it characteristically involves creases of skin such as the bend of the elbow, the backs of the knees, the wrists, earlobes, eyelids, and often the neck and face. In fact, it may involve the whole body. The lesions tend to be dry, brownish-gray, scaly, and thickened. The thickened skin shows accentuated skin markings and there is intense, almost unbearable itching.

In infants and young children, certain foods will sometimes provoke attacks of atopic dermatitis. Offending foods include cow's milk, eggs, fish, wheat, and peanuts. In older persons, food allergy is unlikely to be the cause of atopic dermatitis.

Individuals with atopic dermatitis should be under the treatment of a dermatologist. Atopic individuals should avoid 1) rapid changes in temperatures, 2) any violent exercise that provokes sweating, 3) rough, scratchy, tight clothing, especially woolens, 4) frequent use of soaps, hot water, and other cleansing procedures that tend to remove natural oil from the skin, and 5) emotional upsets. These stimuli will provoke itching. Your dermatologist can usually help you by prescribing external and internal remedies to control the itching.

Patients with atopic dermatitis are very susceptible to severe infections with certain viruses such as herpes simplex. The lesions of atopic dermatitis are prone to infections with *Staphylococcus aureus*. Patients with atopy are especially likely to develop severe reactions to injections of penicillin, foreign sera, and certain other drugs.

Sometimes a radical change in environment helps. Many individuals do well when they leave a damp climate with wide variations in temperature and move to a warm, dry climate. However, a few fare better in warm, humid regions. You can obtain more information on atopic dermatitis by writing to the American Academy of Dermatology.

17

Insects and Bugs

Bee and Wasp Stings

What's the best treatment for bee sting? Any tips on how to avoid bees?

Wasp and bee stings are so common that most people know about them. Intense burning and pain occur, followed immediately by itching and swelling.

Bees can leave their stinger and the attached venom sac well anchored in the skin, so it's important to remove both as soon as possible without putting pressure on the sac. The wasp removes its stinger so it can sting again. Local reactions to bee and wasp stings last a few hours and are confined to an area an inch or so in diameter. However, a generalized and potentially life-threatening reaction occurs in about 2% of those stung. This reaction involves abnormal swelling, massive hives, wheezing and difficulty breathing, diarrhea, a drop in blood pressure, shock, and occasionally even death. Prompt attention by a physician is mandatory. Desensitization of the sensitive person with "allergy shots" may be advisable, and the extremely sensitive patient should carry a kit containing antihistamines and epinephrine as prescribed by their physician whenever outdoor activities are planned.

For mild, local reactions, calamine lotion, a cool compress or an ice bag, and an antihistamine are helpful. If swelling exists, epinephrine may be indicated. Apply a tourniquet if possible.

There are several ways to help protect yourself from bees. Wear white or light-colored clothes instead of dark colors, which may attract or antagonize bees. Avoid using perfumes, hairspray, hair tonic, suntan lotions, and similar cosmetics because bees are attracted by their odor. Always wear shoes outdoors. People who have severe allergies to bee stings can also wear protective nets when they are near bees—or run the risk of being stung.

Chiggers

What's the best treatment for chigger bites?

Chiggers (harvest mites) are the American red bugs, which are widely distributed throughout the United States. The mites do not burrow, and they will fall off without treatment. However, within a few hours after chigger bites, itching, redness, and hives appear. Blisters can follow and discomfort is intense.

Good mosquito repellents sprayed on the exposed skin and clothing provide the best protection. The more effective repellents include N,N-diethyltoluamide (deet), dimethyl carbate, and benzyl benzoate. Powdered sulfur has also been used. Check the label of any repellent you plan to purchase to determine whether it contains any of these chemicals.

If you are bitten by chiggers, bathe as soon as possible to help remove them from the skin. Cooling lotions, such as calamine, and cool compresses may help relieve itching and irritation. Physicians may prescribe antihistamines and topical and/or oral steroids for more severe cases.

Insect Repellents

What should I look for in an insect repellent? Which is best for mosquitoes?

Insect repellents work well against mosquitoes, chiggers, ticks, fleas, and varieties of biting flies. They don't work against bees, wasps, and ants.

The most effective active ingredient is a chemical called N,N-diethyltoluamide (deet). Most insect repellents today contain this ingredient, but some contain 2-ethyl-1,3 hexanediol (Rutgers 612), which is slightly less effective. A few products contain both. Other active ingredients such as dimethyl phthalate (DMP) may also be included in some products. DMP is supposed to enhance protection against ticks and chiggers.

Products that contain deet work better and longer than those that contain Rutgers 612. The concentration of deet in commercial products ranges from 5 to 100%. The higher the concentration of repellent, the longer the repellent works, but it's usually not necessary to use a product with more than 50 to 55% deet, except in extreme circumstances.

The maximum-strength products containing 100% deet are more apt to feel uncomfortably sticky or oily and to produce skin irritation. They are also more difficult to apply thinly and evenly to the skin.

As little repellent as possible should be applied to the skin, because the products may cause skin irritation. And don't get repellent in the eyes or on the lips. You may want to try a patch test first to be sure you can tolerate a particular product. You can do this by applying a small amount to your forearm. Check the spot for redness and irritation over the next 24 to 48 hours. If no redness develops you can safely use the product.

Repellents should not be used on small children unless exposure to insects is intense. Then a product with the lowest effective concentration of deet should be used.

Swimming, other physical activity, and perspiration will dilute or rub off the repellent, so it must be reapplied periodically. Generally, repellents with lower concentrations of deet have to be reapplied every hour or two.

Repellents should be applied to both clothing and skin for maximum protection. Mosquitoes can bite right through lightweight clothing such as T-shirts.

Repellents can be applied safely to cotton, wool, and nylon but may damage other fabrics, especially synthetics. They will also damage plastic and painted surfaces. So be sure to keep repellent away from watch crystals and eyeglass frames.

Spiders in Bed

I found a spider in my bed and I'm afraid of being bitten. Are all spider bites dangerous?

The sight of a spider in bed arouses extraordinary fear in most people—but spiders rarely bite humans. Except for those of highly venomous species (for example, black widow spiders, brown recluse spiders, or scorpions), most spider bites are minor problems.

Usually the reaction is a sharp, stinging pain with a swollen, red, hivelike area developing around the puncture wound. In more sensitive individuals, a larger palm-sized area of redness may develop around the bite. Symptomatic treatment with ice packs, calamine lotion, and antihistamines is helpful; cortisone pills or injections hasten recovery.

Brown Recluse Spiders

I've heard it's dangerous to be bitten by the brown recluse spider. What happens?

The venom of the small brown house (recluse) spider (*Laxosceles reclusa*) destroys the skin at the bite site. The venom can also produce severe internal reactions.

There is no pain after the bite of a brown recluse spider for at least 7 to 8 hours. The first clinical sign is redness, which is followed by a blister, hemorrhage, and eventually an ulcer. Brown recluse spider bites are more common in the southern United States, although such bites have also occurred in the northern states. If you think you have been bitten by a brown recluse spider, you should see your dermatologist or other physician promptly. If necessary, go to the nearest emergency room as soon as possible for diagnosis, evaluation, and treatment. Alert the physician that you have been bitten by a spider and, if possible, bring the spider for examination.

The brown recluse spider is easily identified by the light spot on its back that resembles a fiddle, thus the common name fiddle-back spider.

Bedbugs

I worry about bedbugs. What do bedbug bites look like? How do you treat them?

Bedbugs are most often found in older and poorly maintained buildings. They require warmth. They usually feed at night; during the day they usually hide in crevices, furniture, and loose flooring.

Most people sleep through the biting attack but find the hivelike skin changes, blood, and scratch marks in the morning. In a highly sensitive individual, the hivelike spots may last several weeks and be very itchy. They are usually grouped close together, and frequently occur in a line. Old lesions can be reactivated by new bites.

The bites are treated symptomatically with applications of cool compresses or an ice bag. Your physician may prescribe antihistamine drugs or topical steroids to help resolve the rash. The source of the pests must be controlled by chemicals and their daytime hiding areas eliminated.

Pediculosis pubis (Crabs)

What causes crabs? What's the best treatment?

The pubic, or "crab," louse (*Phithirius pubis*) is usually contracted during sexual intercourse but can be picked up from contaminated bedding, toilets, clothing, etc. They may be found in any hairy area (including the eyelashes), but are usually found only in the genital area unless the individual is heavily infested. They cling to the hair or on the adjacent skin at the base of the hairs, and appear as grayish scales.

The nits (eggs) are attached to the hairs just above the skin. Finding the nits or the louse establishes the diagnosis. Dried, bloody crusts may also be noted on the skin or in the underwear or the pajamas. These are the result of scratching and help establish the diagnosis.

Lindane-containing preparations, applied topically, are usually prescribed by physicians for treatment. A new product, permethrin, is also very effective. Synthetic pyrethrins available as over-the-counter products are generally effective for treatment. Sexual contacts should be examined and treated as indicated.

Clothing and linens should be washed or dry-cleaned. Clothing that has not been worn for at least two weeks can be considered safe because the lice will die in that time period.

Since *Pediculosis pubis* is usually transmitted through sexual contact, it may be appropriate to check for other sexually transmitted diseases, depending on the individual's history.

Head Lice

My daughter caught head lice at school and I'm furious. Is this common?

It certainly is. Studies show that three to five children in a hundred, in almost every elementary school in this country, are infested with head lice. Adults are also susceptible to lice, but white schoolchildren are the most frequent targets (black children are rarely affected). Children of all social and economic levels can be infested.

Intense itching of the scalp is the primary symptom of lice infestation. The back of the scalp is usually the most affected area. Because of the itching, there are likely to be many scratch marks and secondary infection is common. There may be enlarged lymph glands in the neck. The nits (eggs), which are white and oval, are attached to the hairs. The nits may appear to be flakes of dandruff, but they cannot be dislodged by brushing. When a metal comb is used, there is a clicking sensation as the comb strikes the nits. The adult lice, which reside on the scalp, are about the size of sesame seeds and are more difficult to see.

Fortunately, effective, relatively simple treatment is available. The most widely used treatment involves the use of a special medicated shampoo containing lindane, as prescribed by a physician. Since there is some concern about the safety of lindane in very young children, other products are often used. Many of these contain pyrethrins, benzyl benzoate, and sulfur. The nits should be removed by combing with a fine-toothed comb. Treatment should be repeated after about 10 days.

Clothes and bed linen should be washed in hot water and dried on the hot cycle. If one member of the family has lice, everyone else should be checked.

Lice may spread from head to head directly or indirectly, via combs, scarves, caps, and bed linen. You should tell your children never to share personal items with schoolmates. All affected children in school should be treated. The school situation can be a public health problem which, in most instances, is very difficult to solve. It becomes very important to deal with the emotional problems associated with this relatively innocuous and innocent, but annoying, condition.

Scabies

What causes scabies?

Scabies is an eruption caused by infestation with the itch mite (*Sarcoptes scabiei* var. *hominis*). It is characterized by severe itching at night. The sites most commonly involved are the finger webs, toes, wrists, outer elbow area, armpits, genitals, nipples, and navel. The head is rarely involved except in infants.

The rash and symptoms are due to sensitization and irritation caused by the female mites, which live and lay their eggs in burrows of the skin. The burrows appear as slightly red, thread-like channels, or "runs." The mite may be visible as a dark speck at one end of the burrow. Scratch marks, small red pimples, and skin irritation are common.

The most commonly used therapeutic agents are 1% lindane cream or lotion, 10% crotonotoluide cream or lotion, benzyl benzoate, and topical sulfur ointments. If there is secondary bacterial infection, topical and oral antibiotics may be necessary. After the mites have been destroyed, the residual annoying rash may last for weeks and require additional treatment. To treat scabies effectively, the source of the problem must be identified. All contacts and those living in the same quarters must be treated at the same time even if there are no symptoms of scabies. Changing bed linens and washing clothing worn at the time are important to prevent re-exposure.

Sand Flies ("No-See-Ums")

On a vacation to the Caribbean, I was bitten by "no-see-ums." What are they?

Sand flies ("no-see-ums") are small blood-sucking insects. These annoying, biting insects frequently meet their prey during the latter's vacation in the southern United States, Caribbean islands, and Mexican beaches. Also known as gnats, sand flies, "biting midgets," and "punkies," they bite the exposed skin of the extremities, the face and neck, and even the scalp. The female fly usually attacks at sundown.

The small, red, itchy bumps that appear after the bites last for hours or days. In more sensitive victims, the itching may be intense and can last for weeks. In these cases, it may be necessary for your physician to prescribe orally administered cortisone-like drugs.

Creeping Eruption

What is creeping eruption?

Creeping eruption is the common name given to an infestation of the skin with larvae of the dog or cat hookworm. The medical term for the disorder is larvamigrans.

It is a common infestation in the southeastern United States in areas contaminated by dog and cat feces. Contact usually occurs on moist sandy soil (children's sandboxes, beaches). Uncovered skin is vulnerable. For this reason, the hands or feet are usually affected, although any area of the skin can be involved. Dozens of spots may occur on a single person.

Right after penetration of the skin by the larvae, minute, itchy, and swollen red bumps (papules) appear. Within 2 to 3 days the characteristic snakelike rash begins as the larvae begin to migrate. If untreated, the lesions may continue to spread for several months. Itching is intense. The disease cannot be spread from one person to another, and eventually the larvae die or are destroyed by the body. Thiabendazole (a prescription drug) is very effective orally and topically.

Fleas

Can my cat's fleas attack me?

Although fleas are primarily parasites of other animals, such as dogs and cats, they may on rare occasions cause problems in humans. This is particularly true if the animal is heavily infested. Flea bites may cause itchy, red bumps, blisters, and even small infected pustules.

A peculiar itchy, hivelike rash occurs primarily on the lower legs and can last days to weeks. It appears most frequently during warm weather. Everyone is susceptible, but children or those in poorer circumstances are more likely to be involved.

The diagnosis may be difficult, but fleas should be suspected if the characteristic rash is present below the knees. This is the usual eruption pattern if animals in the house are not allowed on furniture and beds. It is common for more than one family member to have bites. It is wise to have the animals examined and treated as necessary; often the house has to be fumigated. The skin rash can be treated with calamine lotion, topical corticosteroids, cool compresses, and oral antihistamines. Orally administered cortisonelike drugs prescribed by a physician may be needed in the most severe, resistant cases.

18

Nutrition and the Skin

Vitamins and the Skin

Which vitamin supplements help the skin?

None. Vitamins are part of the total nutritional intake (protein, fats, carbohydrates, minerals) and are essential for normal skin metabolism and physiology. However, there are no vitamin supplements that are especially helpful to skin. As with thyroid and insulin, there is an optimal vitamin dose that should not be exceeded; to do so may invite side effects involving the skin and internal organs.

Nonetheless, vitamin A has been popularly used as "the skin vitamin." Excessive amounts of vitamin A are dangerous and may cause dry and fissured lips and skin, brittle nails, hair loss, and many very dangerous internal changes. Toxicity has been reported with the intake of as little as 15,000 to 25,000 units daily for prolonged periods of time. Birth defects may be associated with very high intake. Vitamins D and K, niacin, and pyridoxine can also be toxic in excessive amounts.

Oily and Greasy Foods

Do oily and greasy foods make the skin more oily?

It is a popular belief that greasy foods and oil make the skin oilier. However, the oily foods we consume do not influence the skin's degree of oiliness.

The "oiliness" of the skin is a perception of the natural emulsion (mixture of oil and water) that covers the skin surface. This results from the mixture of oil (sebum) from the sebaceous glands (the oil glands of the skin) and oil from the cells on the skin surface with the perspiration from the sweat glands. If the humidity is high, the sweat does not evaporate from the skin surface. This is why the skin feels oily or sticky on hot, humid days. The increased intake of fats has no influence on the amount of oil produced by the sebaceous glands, which is under hormonal control.

"Feeding" the Skin and Hair Topically

Can you "feed" skin and hair by applying foods and vitamins to the skin?

No. The hair is a dead structure, unable to use anything that is "fed" to it on the surface. The only living part of hair is deep in the skin. Certain materials may adhere to the hair shaft so the hair *appears* thicker. Some material may even penetrate into the dead hair shaft, but this will not have any effect on hair growth. The effect is limited to temporary "conditioning," like that provided by any conditioner.

While the outermost layer of the skin is composed of dead cells similar to those of the hair, many materials can penetrate through this layer into the living skin and into the circulation. In fact, certain heart and anti-seasickness medications are delivered through the skin very effectively via drug-containing adhesive plasters applied to the skin. However, the implication that one can feed the skin as one does a lawn to replenish minerals, protein, and vitamins is an oversimplification of a complex biological process. The topical application of certain materials may change the skin's chemical or physiological activity, but the product must then be considered a drug, not a cosmetic.

Effect of Diet on the Hair

What effect does diet have on hair?

The hair root is an exquisitely sensitive growing organ. Any severe, systemic insult will traumatize the growing hair and result in premature cessation of growth. The hair then goes into the resting phase of the growth cycle and is shed. Significant dietary changes such as severe, sudden reduction in calories, starvation, or significant protein deficiency may thus result in temporary hair loss. The more severe the dietary insult, the more severe and acute the hair loss.

Fortunately, hair loss of this nature will stop over a period of about three months after a proper diet has been reinstituted. The lost hair is gradually replaced. Similar hair regrowth has occurred in starving prisoners of war.

Protein Deficiencies and the Skin and Hair

Do severe protein deficiencies affect the hair and skin?

The classic example of protein malnutrition is a disease called kwashiorkor, which is characterized by a reddish coloration of the hair, redness and superficial scaling of the skin, and a variety of internal symptoms.

In dark-skinned people, lightening of the skin may appear, primarily around the mouth and on the lower extremities. Whites develop redness of the skin and bruise easily.

Varying degrees of change in the skin occur, ranging from fine scaling and cracking to actual loss of the skin. The hair becomes lighter and thinner and falls out easily. Periods of good and bad nutrition are reflected in the hair as stripes of lighter and darker colors.

Fortunately, such severe protein deprivation occurs rarely in this country and usually reflects cult-type diets. However, in Africa, India, and other areas in which starvation is a problem, signs of protein starvation may be seen.

Vitamin Deficiency and Dry Skin

Can a vitamin deficiency cause dry skin? I heard that taking vitamin A, in particular, would help dry skin.

The primary cause of dry skin in otherwise healthy individuals is loss of moisture from the skin. This subject is discussed in detail in Chapters 7 and 12. Taking vitamin supplements will not prevent or cure the average case of dry skin.

While it is true that severe deficiencies of certain vitamins may have an adverse effect on the skin (as well as other organs), such deficiencies occur only in starvation, severely restricted diets such as fad diets, or various medical disorders. All these conditions require medical consultation, and a physician will prescribe the necessary vitamins and proper nutritional counseling.

It is a common misconception that dry skin results from a deficiency of vitamin A as it is frequently referred to as "the skin vitamin." However, no such relationship exists. In fact, too much vitamin A is toxic; therefore, you should never take supplements containing high dosages of vitamins unless your physician has determined that you have a true deficiency.

No one is going to be harmed by taking a daily multivitamin, but other vitamin supplements are generally unnecessary unless prescribed by a physician for a specific problem.

19

Miscellaneous
Skin Problems

Pregnancy and the Skin

What skin changes can I expect during pregnancy? Are any special skin care measures recommended?

Pregnancy produces many changes in the body, including in the skin. Hair and nails usually grow faster than normal. The body becomes warmer, so pregnant women tend to perspire more. This problem can be controlled with deodorant and antiperspirants, frequent showers, and wearing loose, comfortable clothing.

As the skin stretches over the abdomen to accommodate the growing fetus, stretch marks (striae) may appear. Application of emollient creams and lotions can make the stretched skin feel more comfortable, but there is no way to prevent stretch marks.

Pigmentation also changes during pregnancy. The nipples darken, and some women develop a vertical brown line in the middle of the lower abdomen that slowly lengthens toward the belly button as the uterus enlarges. Pigmented moles, freckles, and birthmarks also tend to become darker, and increased pigmentation called melasma or the "mask of pregnancy" may appear on the forehead, cheeks, or elsewhere (see Chapter 26 for more details on melasma).

Due to the growth of new small blood vessels, lesions called spider angiomas may appear as red spots or spiderlike tracings anywhere on the skin, and streaks may appear on the abdomen or thighs. The veins on the legs often become prominent and tortuous. Many women are bothered with varicose veins and hemorrhoids, especially in the later stages of pregnancy.

Itching is another common problem complicating pregnancy. This can usually be relieved with soothing creams or lotions applied several times a day. Baths in tepid water to which colloidal oatmeal has been added also relieve itching. However, if itching is severe or prolonged, you should consult your physician.

Some chronic skin problems such as acne, eczema, and psoriasis may also be affected by pregnancy. Usually the conditions improve, but sometimes they worsen.

Most of these changes are within the normal range and should not be cause for any special concern. Most disappear within a month or two after childbirth. The exception is stretch marks. While they may gradually fade over time, they never totally disappear. Surgery to remove stretch marks remains controversial.

One problem that may occur within the first few months after giving birth is temporary hair loss. See Chapter 3 for more information on this subject.

Infant Skin Care

What special precautions should be observed in caring for the skin of a newborn infant? What are common skin problems parents can anticipate?

The skin of a newborn is not fully formed or functional. It is thin and is not a good protective barrier. The sweat glands, oil glands, and hair follicles also may not be fully developed. Thus, an infant's skin is more delicate and more easily harmed by things that come in contact with it. In addition, some skin problems are especially common in the infant due to this incomplete development.

Keep an infant out of the sun; even moderate exposure may cause a severe sunburn. Avoid contact with hot water or other hot liquids, as an infant's skin is easily burned. Chemicals, medications, or other products can easily penetrate the skin and cause allergies or other problems. Don't apply anything to infant skin unless your physician has approved its use.

Since the sweat ducts tend to become easily blocked in infants, they may develop prickly heat when the air is warm and humid.

Infants may also develop a rash (intertrigo) in skin folds due to moisture retention when the temperature and humidity are high. Intertrigo occurs when moisture and friction cause irritation and redness of the opposing surfaces of the skin in the folds. If yeast or bacteria invade the area, medical attention may be necessary. Mild cases of prickly heat and intertrigo can usually be cured by regulating the temperature and humidity, dressing the infant in loose, cooler clothing, and avoiding the use of greasy ointments. It is helpful to periodically wipe the skin with a cool, damp sponge or soft washcloth.

The scalp hair that is present at birth is usually shed within a few weeks, and it may take several months for the scalp to once again be covered with hair.

Diaper rash, the other extremely common skin problem that afflicts infants, is discussed in the following question and answer.

Diaper Rash

What's the best way to prevent diaper rash? What treatment is recommended when it does occur?

Diaper rash is so common that most infants suffer from it at least once. It is an inflammatory skin reaction that appears on areas covered with diapers—the buttocks, genital area, upper thighs, and lower abdomen. The skin becomes red and raw; pimples and bumps may appear on the red areas.

A combination of factors are involved in producing diaper rash. Prolonged contact with urine damages the skin barrier, producing irritation. Bacteria in the feces break down chemical wastes in the urine, causing more irritation. Once irritation is present and the outer layer of the skin is damaged, the skin is more susceptible and the rash worsens. Certain bacteria and yeast may take advantage of the moisture and the food supply available in feces to produce a superinfection.

The best way to avoid diaper rash is to change diapers frequently and to gently cleanse the skin to remove feces with *every* diaper change. Be sure to rinse thoroughly and gently wipe dry. You don't want to further irritate the skin. Then apply mild ointment or cream. Diapers must be smooth, soft, and clean.

If diaper rash occurs, be even more diligent about changing diapers. Change them every hour if necessary. Don't ever change diapers without gently cleansing, rinsing, and drying the diaper area. If possible, avoid the use of disposable diapers and rubber or plastic pants. Let the baby go without any diaper in warm weather, if practical.

If these measures are not successful and diaper rash persists for more than a few days, consult your physician. It may be necessary to prescribe medications such as steroids and/or antibacterial preparations.

Skin Care in the Elderly

What are the special skin-care needs of the elderly?

This is a tremendously important area of skin care. The elderly have special needs because their skin is thinner and drier. Efforts should be made to keep the skin from becoming even drier. The frequency of bathing and showering should be reduced. Use warm rather than hot water. Exposed areas of the skin should be covered to protect against cold and wind. Regular daily lubrication of the skin, especially the legs, is essential. Itching of the legs in the elderly living in northern climes during late fall or in the early winter is common, so the use of lubricants should be increased to prevent additional dryness.

Low humidity, which increases skin dryness, is common in desert areas, in hot-air-heated homes and air-conditioned environments. Consequently, dry skin problems may appear in southern and desert areas as well as in northern climates.

Those who are sedentary need to reduce pressure on ankles, heels, and the buttocks–sacral area. The skin of the elderly needs the same gentle care one would give the skin of a baby or young child.

Cosmetic skin care in the elderly should be simple, enjoyable, and directed toward minimizing dry skin and improving social and personal acceptance. Good grooming is important psychologically for the elderly. Emotional depression can be seen in the unkempt. It is uplifting to be neat, attractive, and acceptable in society. Most cosmetic and toiletry products (except those that are too drying or irritating) can be used by the elderly.

Care of Scars

What treatment is recommended for scars?

The treatment of scars varies depending on type and location.

Acne scars can be improved by makeup, collagen, and fibril injections, dermabrasion, surgical removal, and deep chemical peels. Treatment must be individualized. Each form of treatment has some limitations in effectiveness.

Scars that form after burns, surgery (e.g., mastectomy scars), and radiation therapy require surveillance. Treatment includes lubrication, avoidance of unnecessary trauma, and immediate care of injuries to the scar. If the last is not done, chronic rashes and ulcers may occur.

Thickened scars (hypertrophic scars, keloids) occur more frequently in blacks. They may appear following minor injuries or after prolonged stimulation of the skin repair process. When healing is prolonged or delayed, or chronic infections occur, a thickened scar can develop. This is seen frequently with large burns and pierced ears. Such scars should be kept lubricated; they may be improved by injecting them with cortisone or by surgical excision or laser removal. Pressure on scars should be avoided for comfort and to prevent pressure ulcers.

Heat, Humidity, and the Skin

How is the skin affected by heat and humidity?

The skin is remarkable in how well it adjusts to wide variations in temperature and humidity, but increased heat and humidity may exacerbate various skin conditions. The obvious initial response to elevation in both heat and humidity is increased sweating.

Sweating may increase itching and burning in many skin conditions. Prolonged heat and humidity increase the incidence of rashes in skin creases, fungus infections, prickly heat, and bacterial infections. Problems such as eczema are aggravated by sweating. Also, when exercise programs—which are increasing in popularity—are performed in hot, humid environments, the sweating (and sometimes friction) will exacerbate acne and can lead to problems with body heat regulation.

In tropical climates, increased sweating is almost constant. The skin seems damp and oily, and is more prone to low-grade infection.

Prolonged sweating may lead to soggy skin and increased foot odor. Underarm odor may also be increased. Heat and humidity may also cause an increase in dermatitis in the genital and axillary areas, particularly in obese individuals.

Care revolves around frequent cleansing (bathing, showering), the use of antiperspirants and deodorants, and frequent changes of clothing and shoes.

Telangiectasia and Varicosities of the Legs

What causes reddish-blue streaks of discoloration on the legs?

The tortuous, linear, and threadlike red to blue discolorations are dilated veins and capillaries. They are more common in women, starting in young to middle age. They tend to increase gradually. The broken capillaries are called telangiectases; larger varicosities may become varicose veins.

Such varicosities are aggravated by pregnancy, prolonged standing, and other activities that increase venous pressure in the lower extremities. Wearing support hose and avoiding aggravating activities are important elements in their management.

Treatments include covering with makeup, destruction by electrolysis or laser therapy, and injection of individual veins with saline (salt water) or other irritating chemicals. However, treatment can lead to superficial scarring or brown staining. The discoloration can last from months to several years.

Cayenne Pepper Spots (Red Spots)

What are cayenne pepper spots?

These red spots are also known as senile hemangiomas, cherry spots, and ruby spots. They are small, raised, smooth, red or purple papules found primarily on middle-aged and older persons.

Such spots have no known relationship to medical problems. The lesions sometimes become very dark, causing concern about skin cancer. Removal for cosmetic reasons can be done easily by electrocautery or other destructive measures.

Emotional Stress and Skin Problems

Can emotional stress cause skin problems?

Emotional stress, while very influential in the course of many skin problems, is not usually the primary cause of disease. It is often impossible to identify a direct cause-effect relationship between an emotional reaction and a specific skin disease.

Emotional factors, however, have been linked to excessive sweating, localized eczema, itching, neurotic excoriations, flushing, and other problems. Many cases of hives are undoubtedly the direct result of significant psychological stress. More severe and deep-seated problems are associated with self-inflicted skin disorders that serve to bring attention to the individual, help collect insurance, or permit the person to avoid combat service. Other conditions related to emotional conditions include hair-pulling (trichotillomania), neurotic picking and scratching, and delusions of parasitosis (excoriations to rid skin of imagined parasites). Those with the last affliction are severely disturbed and need psychiatric help.

Increased sweating of the palms, soles, and underarms is primarily a response to emotional stress. Cold, wet hands are a cause of embarrassment for many people. Topical care, oral medications, and emotional support help. Surgery is an alternative for severe underarm sweating. See Chapter 15 for a detailed discussion of perspiration problems.

Perhaps the greatest psychiatric component of skin diseases is the stress placed on the individual who has socially unacceptable skin and hair changes. This can lower the individual's self-esteem and affect relationships with others. From the high school teenager with acne to the newlywed with severe psoriasis or eczema to the adult woman with little scalp hair, one can see the gamut of those experiencing stress as they try to get along in a world in which their appearance may be unacceptable.

Closing the Pores

I have often heard people say that a hot shower followed by a cold one will close the pores of your skin. Is it possible to close the pores? Is it true that a hot shower should be followed by a cold one to close the pores?

There is no scientific basis for this claim. The visible pores on the skin's surface are the openings of the hair and oil gland follicles. The sweat glands also open on the surface of the skin through pores but are visible only with a magnifying lens. The size of all of these pores cannot be altered, nor can they be opened and closed.

When you take a hot bath or shower, the heat may increase circulation slightly by causing small blood vessels close to the skin surface to dilate. A cold shower immediately afterward will constrict the blood vessels and may feel good, but it serves no other purpose.

Food Allergies and Skin

Can food allergies cause skin rashes?

Food allergies and skin rashes have been linked for many years, but the connection between the two is greatly overemphasized. The skin problems most commonly thought to be associated with food are acne vulgaris (probably unimportant, and discussed elsewhere), hives, eczema (atopic dermatitis), and hand eczemas. Hives can be caused by a variety of foods, including shellfish, nuts, and many fruits. The history of an outbreak after eating a particular food is the most important piece of evidence linking foods (their breakdown products or some component) to skin disease.

Some controversy exists over the correlation between food intake and eczema (atopic dermatitis). Perhaps the relationship is more important in infants. Only provocation by actually eating the food helps to establish the relationship.

In addition to reactions from consumed foods, allergic skin reactions from handling foods are also well documented. This problem is experienced primarily by food handlers, housewives, and chefs. In addition, chemicals in foods, or chemicals used to treat foods, can make the skin more sensitive to sunlight.

The best treatment for a *proven* food allergy is to eliminate the food from the diet or, in the case of a contact reaction, to avoid direct contact with the food. Specific treatment may be prescribed by your dermatologist. Desensitization is rarely, if ever, successful.

Cysts

What causes cysts? What treatment is recommended?

A cyst is a noninflamed sac within the skin that contains tissue fluid, cells, and cell debris. It may result from trauma to hair follicles or from pieces of skin buried beneath the surface. There may be a small opening in the cyst through which the contents drain. The size may vary from a pinhead-sized bump to a large lump. Cysts are usually painless unless they become infected or rupture, in which case they resemble boils.

Cysts are harmless and do not require treatment except for cosmetic reasons or unless they become repeatedly infected. It's a good idea, however, to have a suspected cyst examined by a physician since enlarged lymph glands, skin cancers, and other conditions may have a similar appearance.

Boils

What causes boils? What treatment is recommended? Is it okay to squeeze a boil to bring it to a head?

A boil is a tender, hot, red mass, which usually has a small central white or draining area. The material that drains from a boil is a mixture of bacteria, cells, and tissues that have been destroyed in the inflammatory reaction. Boils are infections of the skin caused by pus-forming bacteria (staphylococci). They usually start in hair follicles.

People who suffer from recurrent boils should consult a physician as they may have an underlying disease such as diabetes that predisposes them to infection.

Don't squeeze boils because this may spread the infection. If a boil is painful and does not drain, consult a physician. The physician may incise it to promote drainage, but you should not try to do this yourself.

Treatment of acute conditions should include the use of warm compresses for 10 to 15 minutes at least four times a day. A physician may also prescribe antibiotics.

An important part of therapy is preventing the appearance of new boils. You should take a shower with an antibacterial soap twice a day. When boils recur frequently, underclothing and bed linens should be changed daily. When boils are present, towels, washcloths, and other personal articles should not be shared.

Seborrheic Keratoses

What are seborrheic keratoses? What treatment is recommended?

Seborrheic keratoses are very common warty growths of the outer layer of the skin (the epidermis). Seborrheic keratoses are rough, scaly, raised, greasy-looking growths that vary greatly in size and appearance. They may be smaller than a dime or larger than a quarter. The color may vary from yellow or tan to brown and black. Sometimes they are mistaken for warts or even skin cancers. Seborrheic keratoses occur more frequently from middle age onward and increase in size and number over the years. They occur primarily on the trunk but are also fairly common on the face.

Seborrheic keratoses do not require treatment unless they are being irritated or are a cosmetic problem. They can easily be removed by your dermatologist.

Safe Ear Piercing

I plan to have my ears pierced. Can I have this done in a jewelry store or should I have it done by a physician?

You should have your ears pierced by a physician to minimize potential complications. Instruments used for piercing must be sterile, and proper precautions should be followed during the healing process. Serious infections such as hepatitis and AIDS can be contracted if you have your ears pierced under unsterile conditions.

It only takes a physician a few minutes to pierce ears, and the technique is relatively painless. The first step is to carefully measure and mark the ears because both ears may not be exactly alike. The ears are then pierced with a sterile needle or other instrument, and "starter" earrings or metallic wires are inserted. These starter earrings must be worn for three to four weeks until the wounds heal. They should not be removed before this time unless the area becomes infected or for other medical reasons. New earrings should not be inserted until the wounds are completely healed.

During this critical period, your physician's instructions should be carefully followed to prevent infections or closure of the opening. Once the opening is established it will remain for life, unless irritation or infection results in closure.

If there is any type of rash on the ears, or small cysts in the ears, they should not be pierced. Also, if there is a family or personal history of keloids (scar overgrowth), the ears should not be pierced.

You should avoid earrings that contain nickel, a metal that causes allergic skin reactions more frequently than other metals used for jewelry (see the question and answer on reactions to jewelry in Chapter 16). Once you have become sensitive to nickel, the sensitivity is permanent and your skin will react whenever it comes in contact with nickel again. Sterling silver does not contain nickel and rarely causes allergic reactions; neither does gold if it is 18 karat or heavier. Stainless steel posts are also safe for pierced ears. White gold and German silver contain nickel and are known to cause reactions in nickel-sensitive persons. Most cheap costume jewelry earrings are likely to contain nickel to harden the metal.

Tattoo Removal

What methods are available for the removal of tattoos?

Tattoos may be removed by various methods, but none is completely satisfactory because the pigment in a tattoo extends very deep into the skin. A scar will usually result from any method of removal.

Small tattoos can often be removed by one or more surgical excisions, leaving minimal scarring. Larger tattoos do not lend themselves as well to surgical excision, but a modified surgical procedure will produce superficial scars that may obliterate pictures and names enough to disguise the original tattoo.

Dermabrasion (skin planing), a technique in which the upper layers of the skin are removed, has severe limitations for tattoo removal because the pigments are deposited so deep in the skin that it is necessary to carry the skin removal deep enough to produce scars. A modification of dermabrasion known as superficial dermabrasion has proved successful in some cases. In superficial dermabrasion, the skin over the tattooed area is lightly dermabraded until it becomes irritated. This leads to an inflammatory reaction that causes certain cells to pick up the tattoo pigment and work their way to the skin surface. The tattoo pigments are sloughed off with the cells. In some cases, one treatment may be sufficient to remove the tattoo pigment. In other cases, additional treatments are required.

Salabrasion is a technique that utilizes salt to abrade the skin and set up an inflammatory response similar to that in superficial dermabrasion.

In recent years, laser therapy has been used in many medical applications, including tattoo removal. The laser is a form of intense light, and some of the colored pigments in tattoos are destroyed by this light. The ruby carbon dioxide and argon lasers are used for the treatment of tattoos. If the tattoo is very large, several treatments may be required. Scarring will follow.

Tattooing flesh-colored pigment over the original tattoo is often not satisfactory since it is impossible to completely cover dark blue–black pigments with flesh-colored pigments. Furthermore, tattooed areas may contrast undesirably with tanned skin because the tattooed areas will not tan. It also requires considerable skill to match the pigments.

The person who has a tattoo removed will almost always be left with scarring or another defect. Thus, he or she must decide which is preferable, the tattoo or the defect that remains after treatment. If the decision is made to remove the tattoo, a physician experienced in dermatological surgery should be consulted. The physician will decide if there is a preferable treatment depending on the size and location of the tattoo and other factors.

pH of Skin-Care Products

I understand the skin has an acid pH, so products applied to the skin should be acidic or pH-balanced.

The basis for concern about pH followed the discovery that the skin usually has a slightly acid pH. Fortunately, the skin's buffering capabilities are so great that it can adjust to the variations in the many outside forces that can influence the acidity or alkalinity of the skin surface. It's extraordinary that the skin, with its exposure to almost unlimited external forces, can efficiently adjust its pH to the normal range.

The acid-base balance story has been promoted for medical preparations such as creams and cleansers, and then for consumer products. Much has been made of the pH of various cosmetics. Only prolonged contact with undiluted high- or low-pH compounds will irritate the skin or damage the hair. Examples are sodium hydroxide in hair straighteners and high-pH washing solutions. If used properly, even these can be used by almost everyone without problems. Therefore, in general, the pH factor is not a significant issue in the safety of most cosmetic formulations.

Wart Viruses and Cancer

Are warts associated with cancer?

Over 40 different types of wart virus (human papilloma virus) have been identified. Six of these types of wart virus have been associated with malignancies. However, the circumstances under which warts become malignant are very rare.

The special circumstances under which the wart virus can be associated with malignancy include: 1) warts in newborns, which may be associated with laryngeal papillomas and cancer of the voicebox, 2) cancer of the cervix, 3) low-grade cancer of the penis, and 4) a rare skin condition known as epidermodysplasia verruciformia.

Warts and Immunosuppression

Are warts a special problem for immunosuppressed people?

Yes, warts may present problems for the immunocompromised patient. In a world where immunity is commonly reduced in those treated for malignancies, transplant surgery patients, and those with diseases such as AIDS, warts tend to be multiple and more difficult to eradicate.

Furthermore, multiple warts can indicate that there is a defect in the immune process, although most often that is not the situation.

Special Warts

Please discuss plantar warts and warts in other special places.

Plantar warts, as their name indicates, occur on the soles. They are often multiple. Tenderness associated with these warts can be a major problem, especially when pressure is applied by walking. This can lead to a change in gait. Contrary to popular belief, plantar warts do not grow more deeply in the skin or around the bones. They appear to grow deep into the skin because they are pressed in by bearing weight. Plantar warts are difficult to eradicate. Treatment should be tailored to minimize scarring and avoid discomfort and disability.

Palmar warts (on the hands) present many of the same problems as plantar warts. Pressure on the warts frequently causes pain. Furthermore, the presence of palmar warts may interfere with function and embarrass those who must shake hands often. If palmar warts are present on both hands, it is preferable to treat one hand at a time so the other hand is available for use.

Vaginal warts present special problems because in moist areas the warts tend to multiply. Recurrences are frequent, even after adequate therapy. Frustration for both the patient and the physician can be considerable because no method exists to determine if any more warts are developing. Anxiety is increased by concern about the association with carcinoma of the cervix and other venereal diseases. Treatment by a knowledgeable dermatologist is important so that the patient can understand what can be accomplished and the complications of treatment. If there are vaginal warts, inspection of the cervix and the entire vagina is important; sometimes painting the suspect areas with dilute acetic acid improves the visibility of small lesions. Vaginal warts are usually transmitted sexually; use of a condom offers significant, but not absolute, protection.

Perianal warts, like vaginal warts, are usually spread sexually. The lower gastrointestinal tract (rectum) should be examined in all cases of perianal warts. The warts are often multiple and itchy, and they are more common in homosexual males. Coexistence of other venereal diseases must be excluded. Sexual molestation should be suspected in very young children.

The general treatment of warts depends on the location, type, and number, and the subject's activities and age. Treatments include surgical removal or destruction (laser, electrosurgery), freezing with liquid nitrogen, application of podophyllin (for genital warts) or acids, and immunotherapy. At the present time, there are no anti-viral drugs that are effective for treating warts in humans.

Water Warts (Molluscum Contagiosum)

What are water warts?

Water warts is a common name for skin lesions known medically as molluscum contagiosum and caused by a virus. Molluscum contagiosum lesions can occur anywhere on the skin and in any age group. They appear as smooth, pearly or waxy skin-colored lesions ranging from the size of a pinhead to large lesions with a dimpled center. They usually have a central core that is hard and can be lifted out with a needle.

Molluscum contagiosum lesions are common in children, wrestlers, and swimmers. When they occur on opposing surfaces such as the armpits and the groin, the lesions tend to be multiple. The lesions, which are commonly spread by sexual contact, can be associated with other venereal problems. Molluscum contagiosum is frequently found on the skin of patients with AIDS.

Individual lesions may be destroyed by freezing with liquid nitrogen, mechanical removal, electrosurgery, and the application of acids. The age of the patient, as well as the number and location of the lesions, is important in determining which treatment should be used.

20

Sports-Related Skin Problems

Swimmer's Ear

What is swimmer's ear?

Swimmer's ear is the label given to the itchy, painful, oozing external ear condition that can follow exposure to water. It may cause acute pain and is often the cause of a chronic itching ear problem. It involves the skin lining of the ear canal. Swimmer's ear develops when water is trapped in the ear canal, causing swelling and the breakdown of the outer layer of skin followed by the growth of microorganisms. It is a bacterial infection, although it was once thought to be a fungus infection.

To prevent swimmer's ear, you must not allow water to become trapped in the ear canal. Wearing earplugs while swimming is helpful. If water does get trapped, try shaking it out by hopping up and down with the head cocked to the side. You can also press the hand gently over the ear to produce slight suction and then release it (much the same as you use a plunger to unclog a toilet). If the ear remains blocked, a nurse or physician should be seen. You should not put cotton swabs or other objects into the ear canal because you may induce injury, including perforation of the eardrum.

Specific treatment includes keeping the ear canal open and dry.

Cultures for microorganisms may be needed to identify organisms so that specific treatment can be selected.

Swimmer's Skin and Hair

What skin and hair problems are associated with swimming?

Swimming subjects the skin and hair to many potential problems. Sunburn is probably the most common reaction from swimming outdoors. Contact dermatitis may also be seen, from the sunscreens and other oils and creams that are commonly applied before or after swimming. The hair tends to become drier after prolonged contact with water followed by evaporation and exposure to sunlight. The hair may also become bleached; blond and white hair might even turn green from pool chemicals (copper sulfate used to control algae and microorganisms).

People swim in all kinds of water: pools, lakes, rivers, the ocean, even swamps and brackish water. Each body of water presents hazards to the skin: microorganisms, algae, microscopic worms (cercariae), plants, coral, sharp rocks and foreign objects, and chemicals (pollutants and treatments).

Swimmer's ear is a common problem (see previous discussion). Athlete's foot infections are also extremely common. A condition known as creeping eruption can occur as a result of inoculation of a parasite found in dog and cat feces deposited on beaches. This is commonly found in the southern states. Eye infections can develop from bacteria picked up in swimming pools. The skin can become white and soggy (macerated) from wet swimsuits. This can lead to secondary fungus infections. Chlorine may make the eyes burn and become red and irritated. Chlorine also causes dryness of the skin and hair. Abrasions from rough pool surfaces and rocks may lead to skin infections if left untreated.

After swimming, always shower or bathe. Apply a moisturizing lotion all over the body to counteract dryness. Shampoo the hair and apply a conditioner. Change into clean, dry clothing. Unusual abrasions and cuts should receive prompt attention. If your hair turns green, see a beautician, who should be able to neutralize the color. If you develop a severe sunburn or other skin problem, see a dermatologist.

Exercise Machines and Acne

Can exercising on Nautilus equipment cause acne?

Back friction from Nautilus activities or other friction-producing exercises may aggravate acne. In oily-skinned and acne-prone people, the friction and sweating cause superficial pustules and "pimples."

To prevent this distressing problem, wear smooth clothing, exercise on a smooth surface, and shower as soon as possible. Over-the-counter topical acne products, particularly those containing benzoyl peroxide or salicylic acid, can help. If the condition is severe, oral antibiotics prescribed by a dermatologist are indicated. Any increased pigmentation that follows inflammation and infection will clear slowly over weeks and months. Mild sun exposure can help clear the eruption.

Buttocks Acne and Folliculitis

I seem to get acnelike pimples on my buttocks after playing tennis on hot, humid days. What causes this?

The buttocks are commonly afflicted with an acnelike eruption due to friction, sweating, and microorganisms. The problem seems to be more common in women.

Jogging, playing tennis, and wearing athletic supporters, girdles, pantyhose, rough clothing, and wet swimsuits are risk factros. Hot, humid weather, the inability to shower soon after activities, and the layering of nonabsorbent materials may precipitate the outbreak.

Prevention involves wearing smooth cotton underclothing, cleansing and drying the area frequently, and avoiding the activities that irritate the skin. Don't sit around in damp, sweaty tennis shorts or bathing suits.

Brown discoloration (pigmentation) may follow the inflammatory reaction and may last for months, leaving the area mottled. Oral antibiotics may be necessary for more severe cases and rapid control. Recurrences are common, so daily prophylactic care is important.

Weightlifting and Stretch Marks

Can weightlifting cause stretch marks?

Yes, weightlifting is often the cause of stretch marks. In weight-lifters, stretch marks are usually found around the armpits but they may also be found on the back and groin areas, particularly in those doing leg lifts. Stretch marks also occur in individuals who do heavy manual labor and are commonly associated with obesity and pregnancy. Hormonal changes due to increased cortisone secretions or the administration of cortisonelike drugs can also produce stretch marks. The onset may be insidious or very sudden. Initially, the marks are red or purple but eventually they turn white.

Unfortunately, there is no way to remove the marks. Lubricating with lotions, creams, cocoa butter, or vitamin E has no value in prevention or treatment. If one wishes to prevent stretch marks, weightlifting and other such activities must be avoided.

Wrestling and Skin Infections

Why does wrestling cause skin infections?

The close skin-to-skin contact experienced in wrestling increases the risk of transmission of various infections. In fact, small epidemics among wrestlers of impetigo, boils, herpes infections, warts, and molluscum contagiosum have been well documented. Fungus infections, particularly on the scalp, have been transmitted between young combatants.

Wrestlers are prone to develop fungus infections involving the feet and groin secondary to the sweating and friction accompanying the training and actual wrestling. Bacterial (staphycoccal and streptococcal) skin diseases may occur secondarily on abrasions and scratches that occur during wrestling. Good general skin care during training and after skin injuries will help prevent problems or clear them rapidly.

Jogger's Nipples

What are jogger's nipples?

Itching, sensitivity to touch, pain, and inflammation of the nipples may follow the trauma from rubbing of the nipples by a T-shirt, blouse, brassiere, or sweatshirt while jogging, thus the term "jogger's nipples." Sensitivity to touch and pain can be extreme. Covering the nipples with a smooth cloth or dressing can prevent the problem. If severe, treatment by a dermatologist can help resolve the situation.

Irritation from Football Pads

Every fall when I'm playing football my shoulders break out. What causes this problem?

The problem is due to the shoulder pads. The wearing of shoulder pads combined with sweating and intense exercise friction causes irritation of the skin and sometimes even an infection. Existing acne can be aggravated. This is similar to problems secondary to a shirt collar's rubbing the neck on hot, humid days.

If your shoulder pads are old, frayed, or rough, you should request new, smooth pads to help minimize irritation. You should consult your dermatologist for treatment of irritation and acne. If the condition becomes too severe, you may have to stop playing football, at least temporarily, and you don't want that to happen.

Acne and Irritation from Helmet Chinstraps

I'm really having problems with acne and skin irritation under my football helmet wherever there is friction, especially under my chinstrap. Does the weather (August) have any influence?

Acne may be aggravated in areas where the skin comes in contact with the helmet strap, especially on the chin. The sides of the face and the forehead may also be affected.The causative factors are the same as with shoulder pads, discussed in the previous answer. The heat and humidity that are common in August when practice begins may aggravate the problem.

If your chinstrap is old and rough, try to get a better one. Keep the skin as clean as possible. Consult your dermatologist about other treatment measures.

Jock Itch

What causes jock itch?

Jock itch (intertrigo of the groin) results singularly or in combination with the action of friction, moisture, and fungi. It is more apt to occur in those who are overweight and those who participate in physical activities. If a fungus organism is isolated, it is usually the same fungus that causes athlete's foot. Bacteria may also contribute to the problem.

To prevent jock itch, wear loose clothing, use dusting powder to reduce the friction, and keep the area dry. If the irritation does not respond to preventive measures, or if there is uncomfortable itching and burning, consult a dermatologist to get relief. The dermatologist may prescribe topical antifungal/anti-inflammatory agents. If there is no response, oral drugs may be used.

Petechiae from Exercise

I have developed tiny red spots under my skin that my doctor says are petechiae caused by exercise. Please explain.

Petechiae are a form of purpura, a condition in which tiny hemorrhages occur under the skin. Petechiae appear as pinpoint spots of bleeding. They most commonly affect the feet and legs. There are no symptoms.

The bleeding, which is from the smallest blood vessels, usually follows vigorous exercise carried out while erect (running, weightlifting). Similar changes may appear on the eyelids and the upper arms after activities such as weightlifting, which increases the blood pressure. They can also occur after vomiting, coughing, and sneezing. Some medications—aspirin, for example—increase the likelihood of developing petechiae. Exposure to the sun while taking certain photosensitizing medications can also cause purpura.

The condition usually resolves spontaneously and without any lasting effects except for some pigmentation. Should this condition be severe and persistent, see a dermatologist for a medical evaluation to exclude serious disorders.

Hemorrhages on the Feet from Sports

The skin on my feet looks as if it's hemorrhaging. Can this be due to sports activities?

Hemorrhages involving the feet are common and usually result from shoe trauma. The most common area of hemorrhage are the ends of the toes or underneath the toenails. The lesions may be red, blue, or black. Foot hemorrhages are especially common in soccer players whose shoes are too tight or too loose, allowing the foot to slide. Hemorrhages are also common in tennis and basketball players, who make many sudden stops. The resultant hemorrhages can cause loss of the nail or a frightening dark color that may be confused with a melanoma. Another type of hemorrhaging that most often occurs on the heels looks like bloody sweat droplets. Small capillaries rupture and leak into the skin in small wormlike shapes. Eventually the hemmorrhages disappear.

Blisters

What can I do to avoid blisters on my feet from my jogging shoes?

Blisters that hurt and interfere with function can occur anywhere, but they are most common on the hands and feet. The blisters develop when the skin has been rubbed enough to separate the outer layer (epidermis) from its supporting layer (dermis). They are usually filled with clear tissue fluid but may be filled with blood if a small blood vessel ruptures into the lesion.

To prevent blisters, wear shoes that fit properly. Never, never walk out of a shoestore wearing shoes that are causing burning pain. New shoes should never have to be "broken in"—they should fit right from the start. Wearing Band-Aids, moleskin, two pairs of socks (to cushion the foot and fill the shoe), powder, and clean, dry socks will prevent most blisters.

If a blister is small and asymptomatic, it can be left unopened. If large and symptomatic, the blister can be drained and, if necessary, loose tissue can be trimmed away. The opened blister can become secondarily infected so an antibiotic cream should be applied. Activities that may aggravate the blisters should be avoided. If symptoms such as swelling or redness are severe, a dermatologist should be consulted. Blood poisoning can occur, requiring prompt medical care with oral antibiotics. Red streaks around the lesion are a signal of blood poisoning.

While recurrent, easy blistering may be due to friction, it can also be related to a genetic predisposition. Anyone with neurological or vascular problems (diabetes mellitus) should respect the seriousness of such injuries and consult a physician early.

Abrasions

Should I be concerned about abrasions?

Abrasions are very common in the sports world. Fortunately, most heal spontaneously if not further traumatized. Large abrasions may cause pain, interfere with function, and become secondarily infected. Avoidance of trauma, use of a topical antibiotic ointment, and sometimes the use of an oral antibiotic are indicated. If the wound is dirty, it should be cleansed very thoroughly to minimize the chance of permanent tattooing and infection. Abrasions heal faster when they are covered with a dressing.

Athlete's Foot

What can be done about athlete's foot?

Athlete's foot usually refers to a dermatitis characterized by soggy, white skin (maceration) with surrounding redness seen in the toe webs, particularly between the fourth and fifth toes. It is often accompanied by itching and is associated with sweating and friction. While it may be more common in athletes, it is by no means restricted to them.

In true athlete's foot there is an accompanying fungus infection, since the predisposing factors to fungus infections and dermatitis of the feet are the same: warmth, friction, and thickening of the dead, callused outer layer of the skin. Many people erroneously believe athlete's foot occurs only between the toes. Fungus infections may also involve the soles and toenails.

Fungus infections of the feet vary in their appearance, from being very dry and scaly to frank whitish maceration to blistering and peeling.

Treatment starts with understanding the problem and taking

preventive measures such as keeping the feet dry, wearing dry shoes and socks, and using antifungal foot powders. Following sports activity, shoes and socks should be removed as soon as possible and the feet thoroughly washed and dried.

Specific fungal infections should be treated. Many excellent over-the-counter treatments are available. However, if relief is not adequate or the condition becomes worse, a dermatologist should be consulted for a broader approach to the problem. A more effective topical approach may be started and oral drugs may be prescribed, if necessary.

21

The Sun and Skin

Suntan Is Out; Pale Skin Is In

Why has the medical profession become so adamant about staying out of the sun?

The medical profession is warning everyone about the dangers of suntanning because of the damage the sun does to the skin. Overexposure to the sun leads to premature aging, a rough, leathery texture, freckle-like spots of brown pigmentation (liver spots or senile freckles), precancerous skin growths (solar or actinic keratoses), and, most important, skin cancer. There has been an alarming increase in the incidence of skin cancer in this country over the last 30 years as tanning has become more fashionable.

At particular risk are those who are of Celtic ancestry who have fair skin and freckles; blond, red, or light brown hair; blue, green, or gray eyes; and who burn easily and tan little if at all.

The ultraviolet rays of the sun are responsible for this damage. Experts initially believed that only the ultraviolet radiation responsible for sunburn (UVB) was dangerous, but now we know that the ultraviolet radiation responsible for tanning (UVA) is also potentially harmful. There is even some evidence that long-range infrared radiation (IR) may also be harmful to the skin. While UVB radiation is most intense at midday (10 A.M. to 2 P.M. Eastern Standard Time; 11 A.M. to 3 P.M. Daylight Saving Time), UVA radiation can do damage all day long.

For the sake of your skin, you should forget about the tanned look and go for the porcelain look that was popular in the Victorian era. When you must be out in the sun, you should wear a sunscreen that will provide protection from both UVB and UVA. These products are discussed elsewhere in this chapter.

Sun and Work

My job requires that I work outdoors in the sun, so it's impossible for me to avoid sun exposure. What do you suggest?

Farmers, sailors, cowboys, laborers, construction workers, lifeguards, sports professionals, and many other individuals have to work outdoors. It is extremely important for these people to protect their skin against the years of exposure to the sun by using a good sunblock and, if possible, an umbrella, and by wearing appropriate clothing, including gloves. From experience, many farmers who do not have cabbed tractors have learned to put an umbrella over their tractor seats and wear wide-brimmed hats, long-sleeved shirts, sometimes gloves, and a sunblock.

With people living longer, and working and spending more recreational time outdoors, protection against the sun must become as much a daily routine as bathing and brushing one's teeth.

Use an effective sunblock (SPF 15 or more) daily. If you are unsure about which one to choose, ask your dermatologist or pharmacist to recommend one that blocks out both UVA and UVB.

Understanding the SPF Numbers on Sunscreens

Please explain the meaning of SPF numbers on sunscreens and how you use them to choose the proper product.

During the last 30 years, it has become evident that overexposure to the sun is dangerous because it produces changes such as premature aging and skin cancer. This led the Food and Drug Administration (FDA) to propose a labeling system for sunscreen products that would indicate the degree of protection from sunburning that an individual could expect from a particular product. The FDA proposed that products that claim to minimize sunburning label their products with an SPF (Sun Protection Factor) number ranging from 2 to 15. The higher the number, the greater the protection. This proposal has never become law, and recently products with much higher SPF numbers have become available, some as high as 50.

To determine from the SPF number the degree of protection you will obtain from a product, you must first know how long you can stay in the sun without any protection before you begin to burn. This is referred to as your minimal erythema dose (MED). If you can stay in the sun 15 minutes before you begin to burn, for example, then using a product with an SPF of 2 should enable you to stay in the sun for 30 minutes before you would burn. SPF 4 would enable you to stay in the sun for one hour, while SPF 15 would allow you to stay in the sun for about 4 hours.

The SPF numbers as originally designed related only to the sun-burning ultraviolet radiation (UVB). Today we are aware that the ultraviolet radiation responsible for tanning (UVA) also damages the skin. Recently concern has been expressed that infrared radiation (IR) also contributes to skin damage. If the ozone layer in the atmosphere becomes depleted, another type of ultraviolet radiation (UVC), which is ordinarily screened out by the ozone layer, will become a concern too.

Products with high SPF numbers (15 or more) often protect the skin from both UVB and UVA radiation, and there are claims that a few of the products protect against infrared radiation. If you want optimal protection from sun damage, you should use a product that provides protection against both UVB and UVA radiation. (Information on sunscreen ingredients and the protection they provide is provided in the following question and answer.)

You should not let the SPF of a sunscreen give you a false sense of security. You must not only thoroughly apply the sunscreen initially but also reapply it frequently to obtain the listed protection since the sunscreen will be diluted or removed by sweating, swimming, towels, sand, etc. Don't take labeling claims on products as the gospel truth; they are based on ideal conditions of use that rarely exist in the real world.

Finally, you must realize that none of the sunscreens currently available is 100% effective. If you stay out in the sun long enough, you will eventually burn, even with the "best" sunscreen.

Sunscreen Ingredients

Which ingredients should I look for in a sunscreen?

Sunscreens fall into two categories: chemical and physical. Chemical sunscreens are further broken down into two categories: those that protect the skin from the sunburning rays (UVB) and those that protect the skin from the tanning rays (UVA).

Chemical sunscreens absorb the ultraviolet radiation so it does not penetrate the skin. Effective chemical sunscreen ingredients for UVB protection include para-aminobenzoic acid (PABA), cinnamates such as ethyl-hexyl p-methoxycinnamate and octyl methoxycinnamate, and salicylates such as homo-methylsalicylate. Some individuals are sensitive to PABA and its derivatives so there is a trend toward PABA-free sunscreens. The benzophenones such as oxybenzophenone are effective against UVA radiation. Usually only those products with an SPF of 10 or more will contain chemical sunscreen ingredients that protect from both UVA and UVB.

Some products contain a physical sunscreen ingredient, such as zinc oxide or titanium dioxide, either alone, or in combination with chemical sunscreen ingredients. Physical sunscreens prevent the sun's rays from reaching the skin by blocking and reflecting ultraviolet radiation rather than absorbing it, as do chemical sunscreens. The physical blocking agents provide protection from UVA, UVB, and infrared rays. While the physical sunscreens are quite effective, they leave a visible film on the skin that some people consider unattractive. They also tend to feel greasy and pick up sand and other materials.

Safe Suntanning?

If I am careful not to get a sunburn while I am tanning, won't that mean that I am not damaging my skin?

Sorry, but there is no safe suntan, no matter how carefully you achieve it. The term "healthy tan" is a misnomer. Tanning is really a defense mechanism of the skin. Upon exposure to sun, the skin produces more pigment to provide extra protection against the sun: a tan.

A tan does offer some protection from further sun damage, but at the same time its presence indicates that there has been some degree of damage. Years later this damage is manifested in the form of wrinkles, leathery texture, blotches, sagging tissue, and possibly skin cancer.

It's obviously impossible to always stay out of the sun, but when you must be outdoors, you should protect your skin. While protection is most important during extensive sun exposure—for example, when you are at the beach or playing tennis or golf—you should also have protection when you stroll during your lunch hour, go out in the sun to shop, or water the lawn. Therefore, whenever you are going to be outdoors, you should wear a sunblock, protective clothing, and a hat.

Tips for Suntanning

I want a suntan even if it does damage my skin. What information can you provide to help me minimize the damage and avoid sunburns?

If you insist on getting a tan, then the following information may help you minimize the damage you do to your skin. However, *remember that tanning does damage the skin and is not recommended by dermatologists.*

Sunburns and tans are produced by ultraviolet radiation (UV) from the sun. The total amount of harmful UV radiation that reaches the skin at any given time is influenced by such factors as the seasons, time of day, conditions of the earth's atmosphere, and proximity to the equator (where the amount of UV light is the greatest because its passage through the atmosphere is shortest). For example, sun worshippers soak up more ultraviolet radiation per hour in Florida than they do in Maine because in the South, which is closer to the equator, about 1½ times as much ultraviolet light reaches the earth's surface as in the North.

Try to avoid a sunburn. Fair-skinned individuals with blond or red hair and blue or green eyes (especially those of Celtic ancestry) burn easily. The darker your skin, the more sun you can tolerate before you burn.

Avoid noonday sun. Your chances of developing a sunburn are greatest in the midday hours when the sun is high in the sky and there is less filtration of ultraviolet light by the atmosphere.

Always wear a sunscreen. Select a product that will enable you to get some tanning but will prevent burning. Reapply the sunscreen at least every two hours, or more frequently if you are swimming or sweating profusely. While many sunscreens are somewhat water-resistant, the protection is often not as good as the labeling may claim.

Remember that you can burn even on cloudy or overcast days. Also, it's easier to burn at high altitudes because there is less atmospheric absorption of ultraviolet rays. Wind tends to increase the adverse effects of ultraviolet radiation.

Clothing for Sun Protection

What clothing gives the best protection from the sun?

Most clothing will provide some protection by absorbing or reflecting ultraviolet radiation. Hats, long-sleeved shirts, gloves (work and golf gloves), pants, socks, and shoes provide excellent protection against the sun. In general, the more tightly woven the fabric, the more protection it offers. A light cotton T-shirt has an SPF of about 7, while cotton denim serves as a complete sunblock.

Wet clothing that clings to the skin and very thin or widely woven materials do not provide good protection. Therefore, wearing a T-shirt while swimming is inadequate. Also, white fabric can transmit a large amount of UV light.

Umbrellas for Sun Protection

Will a beach umbrella protect me from burning?

Beach umbrellas do not provide full protection from the sun because the ultraviolet radiation that produces suntan or sunburn can still bounce off reflective surfaces such as sand and water. You will still need to use an effective sunscreen and wear protective clothing.

Sun Protection for Children

Why is sun protection so important for children? I thought they needed sun exposure to absorb vitamin D.

Children should be protected from overexposure to the sun for the sake of their skin in later life. By the time many children reach adulthood, they have already soaked up enough sun to produce their first skin cancers. It is estimated that protection early in life from excessive sun exposure can prevent about 78% of the total expected lifetime skin damage and the associated risk of skin cancer. Experts warn that one severe sunburn during the first 10 to 20 years of life doubles the risk of developing skin cancer later in life. Parents should protect their children from the sun, starting with the day they take the infant home from the hospital.

You should keep children indoors during the middle of the day, as this is when the sun's rays are strongest. When your children must be outdoors, have them wear sun hats, long-sleeved shirts, and long pants. Choose tightly woven fabrics and double layers when possible. Look for a special sunscreen formulated for use on children; there are now several such brands on the market. Apply the sunscreen to all exposed areas. Sunscreens offer relative, not absolute, protection, so children will still end up with a gradual tan over the course of the summer or a winter vacation even if they wear a sunscreen.

Parents should not be misled into thinking that a good dose of the sunlight is healthy for their children. The argument that children get vitamin D from the sun is often used to justify tanning. However, only a few minutes of sunlight are required for vitamin D formation, and food sources (especially vitamin D-enriched milk) are just as effective.

Fake Tans

I understand there are artificial tanning products that can give me a tanned look without having to go out into the sun. What do you think of these products?

There are two types of artificial tanning products: temporary bronzers and longer-lasting stains.

Bronzers, which are often in the form of a gel, contain color pigments that impart a tan color and are very much like makeup bases. They are washed off at night.

The stains contain such chemicals as dihydroxyacetone (DHA). Unless you are careful to apply an even film, you will end up with a streaked tan. Furthermore, rough skin may pick up more color and look darker than other areas. You must also be sure to thoroughly wash your hands after applying the product or the palms will become too dark. If one application does not provide enough "tan," you can reapply the product after about three hours. Each application deepens the color. Finally, a few people develop a yellowish, jaundiced look rather than a convincing tan. You may want to first test the product on a small area to be sure you will like the color. The color will fade about one month after use has stopped.

Remember, from a dermatologist's point of view, artificial tanning products are better for your skin than a regular tan that requires exposure to damaging ultraviolet light. You must realize, however, that artificial tans differ from regular tans in that they do not provide any protection from sunburning.

What to Do About Sunburns

What is the best treatment for a sunburn? Is there any way to avoid peeling after a sunburn?

A sunburn begins with mild redness that reaches a peak within a few hours. The degree of redness may range from mild to severe. A severe reaction, characterized by extreme tenderness, pain, swelling, and blistering, may be accompanied by fever, chills, and nausea—and in extreme cases by unconsciousness within 12 hours of the overexposure. Much depends on the extent and severity of the burn (redness indicating less damage than blistering).

Unfortunately, there is no quick cure for sunburn, despite claims from some sun cream manufacturers. Home remedies, including wet compresses, tub baths, and soothing lotions, usually provide partial relief. Avoid becoming chilled from loss of body heat from red skin. Avoid products that are likely to be too drying (calamine lotion, for example). Be careful about using commercial sunburn preparations, as they often contain local anesthetics that may produce allergic skin reactions.

If you develop a severe sunburn, consult your dermatologist, who may suggest special ointments or oral medications to reduce swelling and pain and prevent infection.

Peeling always follows a severe sunburn; there is no way to avoid the peeling except to avoid the sunburn.

Tanning Accelerators Questioned

Do tanning accelerators really help you get a faster, safer suntan?

Not according to a study conducted at a leading medical center on two heavily advertised products. In their published report the dermatologists stated, "We do not recommend the use of these products, since their claim of efficacy could not be substantiated."

Tanning accelerators were introduced less than five years ago. Their manufacturers claim that the accelerators help the consumer to achieve a darker tan faster, with less sun exposure, thus producing less skin damage. The products are supposed to be used once daily for at least three days before sun exposure.

The key ingredient in these products is tyrosine, an amino acid essential in the tanning process. Unfortunately, tyrosine applied to the skin surface does not penetrate it, and thus cannot perform the same function as the skin's own tyrosine.

Avoid Suntan Parlors

Advertisements indicate that the tanning booths or beds in suntan parlors provide safer suntans than regular sun exposure. Is this true?

No. All sun exposure, natural or artificial, is potentially dangerous to the skin.

Some tanning salons advertise that they provide "safe" tans because they use sunlamp bulbs that emit mostly UVA, the so-called tanning rays, rather than the short UVB, or sunburn, rays. However, UVA also damages the skin. In fact, long-term use of tanning booths or beds may lead to *more* premature aging and wrinkling than regular suntanning because UVA penetrates deeper into the skin than UVB does.

The onset of these harmful effects is delayed. They include an increased rate of aging of the skin and the development of precancerous and cancerous lesions.

Skiing and the Sun

Why do I get worse sunburns while skiing than during the summer? You would think that the sun would be weaker in the winter.

You can get a severe sunburn while skiing because of the altitude and the reflection of the sun from snow. At high altitudes the sun is more intense because it is not filtered as much by the atmosphere and because there is less particulate matter, such as smoke and smog, to filter or scatter the sun's rays. The sun's radiation is further intensified as it bounces off the snow. Snow reflects up to 80% of the sun's rays.

Be sure to wear a sunblock whenever you are skiing. Give particular attention to the nose and lips. If you ski without a cap, the ears may also be burned. Use a sunblock with a cream base; the base will help to protect the skin from windburn and chapping.

Sun-Related Diseases

Are some diseases caused or aggravated by sun exposure?

Some diseases are. These include herpes simplex (cold sores) and a variety of other skin and metabolic diseases.

Lupus erythematosus is one condition that is characterized by sensitivity to the sun. An individual with lupus erythematosus may experience joint pain and have an unusually severe sunburnlike rash after even a short exposure to the sun.

Another condition, porphyria cutanea tarda, is exacerbated by sun exposure; an abnormal chemical in the bloodstream makes the patient more sensitive to the sun. The skin eruption seen in this disease is characterized by blistering on the back of the hands, darkening of the skin, and overgrowth of facial hair.

An increased reaction to sunlight is also a problem for people taking certain medications, particularly some antibiotics, such as tetracycline and its derivatives. Some of the diuretics used in the treatment of high blood pressure, heart failure, and kidney and liver disease may also cause a photosensitivity reaction. Retinoic acid (tretinoin), a popular prescription acne medication that some women use for aging skin, may cause an increased sensitivity to the sun when it is first used.

Photosensitivity

What causes the skin to become photosensitive? What treatment is recommended?

Skin that has become photosensitive is characterized by an exaggerated response or sensitivity to light. Usually the reaction is triggered by sunlight—both indoors and outdoors, as common window glass does not filter out the rays of sunlight responsible for some photosensitivity reactions. Sometimes reactions are triggered by indoor lights such as fluorescent tubes.

The skin reaction may consist of itching, inflammation (redness), or a rash. Dark spots of hyperpigmentation sometimes occur.

Photosensitizing agents are found in numerous products. The list includes certain medications and foods and a variety of items that come in contact with the skin. Commonly used products that may contain photosensitizers include perfumes and colognes, antibacterial soaps, synthetic detergents, medicated cosmetics, shampoos, antiseptic creams, and aftershave products.

In many cases, it is difficult, if not impossible, to track down the source of photosensitization. Compounding the problem is the fact that once a person is sensitized, he or she may also become sensitized to closely related chemicals.

Individuals who have developed photosensitive reactions must minimize their exposure to sunlight. When sun exposure is unavoidable, they should shield themselves with protective clothing and use a maximum-SPF sunscreen (15 or above). Physical sunblocks containing titanium dioxide or zinc oxide provide the most protection but leave an obvious film that may be undesirable.

Sun Poisoning

I developed sun poisoning from a severe sunburn. Will I have to avoid the sun forever?

If by "sun poisoning" you mean you have become allergic to the sun, it's hard to say whether you will remain allergic forever, or whether the sensitivity will gradually fade. Usually these reactions are chronic and recur indefinitely with further sun exposure. In some cases, however, the reaction disappears spontaneously within two or three years. An allergic reaction may appear as bumps, hives, blisters, or red blotchy areas that occur repeatedly in the same area of skin after each sun exposure. Some reactions to the sun are mediated through mechanisms other than allergy.

It's also possible that your reaction is due not to the sun itself but to an ingredient in some preparation that came in contact with the skin, or to some medication that you took. Certain ingredients in plants, cosmetics, skin lotions, sunscreen preparations, and oral medications are photosensitizers. Photosensitizers cause the skin to break out in a rash or hives when the skin is exposed to sunlight.

Prickly-heat-type eruptions are commonly misdiagnosed as sun poisoning. This occurs frequently when an individual living in a winter climate is transported to a tropical climate in a few hours:

The skin is unable to adjust to the sudden change and miliaria (prickly heat) develops.

You should consult a dermatologist to investigate the exact cause of your reaction.

Solar (Actinic) Keratoses

What are solar (actinic) keratoses? I've heard that they may turn into skin cancers.

Solar or actinic keratoses are scaly growths that result from years of sun exposure. They are considered precancerous; somewhere between 5 and 10% may develop into skin cancers if the lesions are left untreated. Therefore dematologists usually want to treat them. These growths are discussed in detail in Chapter 27.

White Spots on Tanned Skin

I have some white spots that mar my tan. Why don't these spots tan?

White spots on tanned skin are usually due to either a fungus infection called tinea versicolor or a loss of the ability to produce pigment, a condition called vitiligo. In the former instance, the lesions may appear as asymmetrical, pinkish to fawn-colored patches on the untanned skin. Tinea versicolor is usually asymptomatic, but occasionally itching may occur. Tinea versicolor usually occurs primarily on the upper body; it rarely involves the face (for more details, see Chapter 25.)

Vitiligo, which is ordinarily symmetrical on both sides of the body, involves a complete or partial loss of pigment, giving the affected area a flat, white appearance. It is asymptomatic but very distressing cosmetically. Vitiligo can involve the face, the hands, and the feet (areas rarely affected by tinea versicolor). The hair in the affected areas may also become white. (For more details about vitiligo, see Chapter 25.)

Many other skin conditions may also cause loss of pigment in tanned skin. You would have to consult a dermatologist to determine the cause of your white spots.

Sun and Water Sports

What precautions should one observe when participating in water sports out in the sun?

Exposure to the sun while in or on the water for long periods of time increases the damaging effects. One must plan to minimize exposure by finding shade when possible or engaging in these sports early or late in the day. Additionally, a good sunscreen that is not easily washed off should be applied before and during sun exposure. If possible, when you are fishing or boating, wear a long-sleeved shirt, long pants, and a wide-brimmed hat. An umbrella will help, too.

Don't be fooled by a hazy sky or a cooling wind. Both lull one into a false sense of safety . . . and a sunburn may be the result. Also, remember that at high altitudes the sun's intensity is increased, so fishing in mountain waters presents a greater hazard for sun exposure. Reflected light from water, deck surfaces, and sandy beaches also increases sun exposure.

Plan carefully when you are going to be out all day participating in water sports. Take all the necessary supplies so you can cope with all eventualities. On the list: sunscreens, lip balms, long-sleeved shirts and blouses, trousers, umbrellas, and wide-brimmed hats. Towels can be used in many different ways to protect the skin from the sun.

Red Neck from Sun Exposure

The back of my neck has become chronically red. Is this due to the prolonged sun exposure I am subject to as someone who works outdoors?

Red to red-brown areas that develop on the sides and back of the neck, called erythromelanosis, are common signs of chronic sun damage. Frequently, the sun damage gives the neck a rippled, or "turkey-skin," appearance. "Red-necks" is used to refer to those with chronic sun damage (usually applied to blue-collar Southerners). The skin beneath the chin, which doesn't get the same degree of sun exposure, is much lighter—closer to one's normal skin color.

The changes are irreversible and a reliable indication of significant sun damage. Treatment is of no value. All you can do is protect the area with a strong sunblock to minimize further damage.

22

Acne

What Is Acne?

Exactly what *is* acne?

Acne is a disease of special types of follicles of the face, back, and chest. It is characterized by a mixture of noninflamed lesions called blackheads (open comedones), whiteheads (closed comedones), and a variety of inflamed lesions, including papules, pustules, and nodules (pimples, or "zits").

Causes of Acne

Just what causes acne? I've heard lots of different stories.

While the exact cause of acne is unknown, there is considerable information on several of the factors involved in this disease.

Acne develops in special follicles (the sebaceous follicles) that have multiple, large sebaceous (oil) glands, a very small hair, and a widely dilated follicular canal, which is visible on the skin surface as a "pore" of the skin. These follicles are located primarily on the face and, to a lesser extent, on the chest and back. The initial event in the development of acne is an abnormally rapid generation of the cells lining the follicular wall. These cells are normally swept out of the follicle, but in acne the newly generated

The dynamics of acne

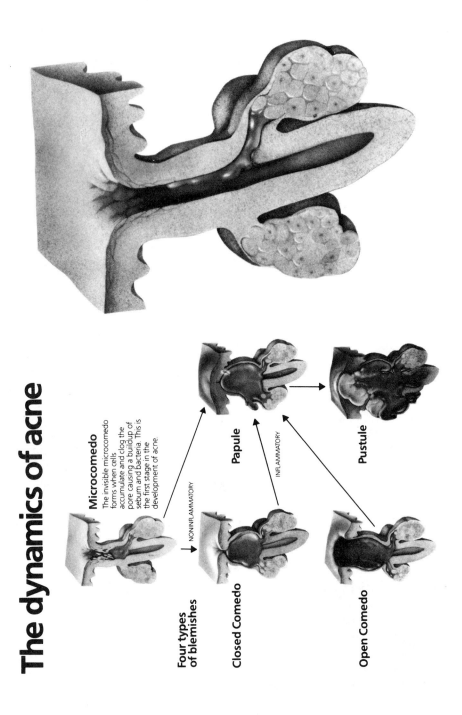

Microcomedo
The invisible microcomedo forms when cells accumulate and clog the pore causing a buildup of sebum and bacteria. This is the first stage in the development of acne.

Four types of blemishes

NONINFLAMMATORY

Closed Comedo

Open Comedo

INFLAMMATORY

Papule

Pustule

cells stick together and form a plug (called a microcomedo) which is invisible from the skin surface. This microcomedo may then enlarge to form a closed comedo (whitehead) or an open comedo (blackhead). In some cases, bacteria in the follicle release products that attract white blood cells (pus) to the follicle. This causes breaks in the follicle wall, leading to more inflammation and pimples (papules and pustules). These sometimes develop into larger lesions called nodules or cysts. (Please see the diagram on page 254 for a clear understanding of the acne process.)

The oily material (sebum) secreted by the skin's sebaceous glands is very important in the generation of acne. Without sebum, acne rarely develops. Acne therefore does not develop before puberty, which is when the sebaceous glands undergo enlargement. The stimulus for the enlargement of the glands is provided by male hormonal substances (androgens), which are found in both men and women.

Sebum itself may play a role in the initiation of the changes in the follicle wall that lead to microcomedos. In addition, bacteria in the follicle, primarily *Propionibacterium acnes*, secrete enzymes that break down parts of sebum into irritating oils called free fatty acids. These fatty acids also stimulate comedo formation. Furthermore, *P. acnes* secretes other products that attract white blood cells, resulting in the inflammatory lesions of acne described above.

Thus, acne is a multifactorial disease that includes increased sebaceous gland activity, follicular hyperkeratosis, and the generation of inflammation by follicular bacteria (*P. acnes*).

Control of Acne

Why isn't there any cure for acne? What is the fastest way to get rid of it? It makes my life miserable.

Acne is a complex disease and, as with many other diseases, the degree of control possible varies. In many cases complete remissions can be obtained; in others only partial control is possible. However, it is not necessary to let acne make your life miserable, and it need not be feared as something that is untreatable. Most cases can be controlled, minimizing the severity and resulting scarring. Left untreated, it can result in permanent scarring and affect your self-image.

The course of acne therapy will vary according to such factors as the type and severity of the case and the patient's age. An individual approach to care and therapy is important in many instances.

Mild cases of acne may respond to the various therapeutic agents you can purchase in a drugstore. These include various special cleansers and topical preparations. They usually contain benzoyl peroxide, sulfur, resorcin, or salicylic acid. Others are abrasives. Many of these treatments are discussed elsewhere in this chapter. If you use one of these products be sure to read and carefully follow the manufacturer's directions for use. If your skin becomes too dry or irritated, use the product less often, or stop using it altogether.

If your acne does not respond to these self-treatment products, you should seek medical treatment from a dermatologist, who will tailor treatment to your specific needs and will most likely prescribe a combination of treatments.

The dermatologist will probably prescribe a variety of topical and oral agents. The most commonly used oral agents are antibiotics. While the dermatologist may remove the closed and open comedones, he or she will most certainly warn you against removing the lesions yourself. This is important because the cells of the follicular wall prevent the contents of the follicle from spilling into the skin and causing inflammation. When you remove the lesions improperly—for example, by squeezing—these natural barriers may be broken down, and more inflammation and scarring may result.

When multiple cysts are present, your dermatologist may inject a corticosteroid preparation into the lesions or drain them.

You must work closely with your dermatologist and follow the recommended treatment regimens. Ask questions if you don't understand some aspect of the treatment program. Together you will be able to control your acne so your life does not have to be miserable.

More information on various acne treatments are found elsewhere in this chapter.

Antibiotics

If acne is not an infection, why do dermatologists prescribe antibiotics? Is it better to take antibiotic pills or to use one of the topical antibiotics you apply to the skin?

Antibiotics are often prescribed for moderate or severe cases of inflammatory acne. They are used to reduce the number of bacteria (*Propionibacterium acnes*) in the follicle (see previous answer on the cause of acne). Antibiotics are not usually prescribed for noninflammatory acne.

Topical antibiotics are usually prescribed for milder cases. Oral antibiotics are usually recommended for more severe, inflammatory acne and resistant cases.

The most commonly prescribed oral antibiotics are tetracycline, erythromycin, and minocycline. If you are taking oral tetracycline you must be sure to take it when your stomach is empty—one to 1½ hours before or at least two hours after a meal. Foods, especially dairy products, interfere with the absorption of the drug from your gastrointestinal tract. So do minerals such as iron in vitamin-mineral mixtures.

Some antibiotics can cause sensitivity to sunlight, so your dermatologist may recommend that you avoid sun exposure and wear a sunblock (a nongreasy formulation). Some people also suffer gastrointestinal upsets and queasiness after taking oral antibiotics during the first few days. Women may develop a vaginal discharge, *Candida albicans*, usually caused by overgrowth of a yeast. This can be treated by your physician, who will advise you as to the best method and whether you can continue to take the antibiotics.

The most commonly prescribed topical antibiotics are erythromycin or clindamycin. These are available in alcoholic solutions, gels, and ointment. Your dermatologist can tell you which preparation is best for your skin.

Benzoyl Peroxide

A lot of acne preparations contain benzoyl peroxide. What does it do? How effective is it?

Benzoyl peroxide is one of the most widely used medications for acne. It is primarily an antibacterial agent, available in over-the-counter products and prescription medications. When applied to the skin, benzoyl peroxide penetrates into the follicles and reduces the population of *Propionibacterium acnes*, the bacterial organism that plays a role in inflammatory acne.

There are some disadvantages to the use of benzoyl peroxide. A few patients may experience mild irritation, and a very small percentage may develop allergic contact dermatitis. Overzealous use may result in excessive dryness. Care must be taken not to get benzoyl peroxide on the hair or on clothing or towels as it may bleach them.

Benzoyl peroxide is available in gels, creams, lotions, masks, and cleansers. Most of the gels must be prescribed by a physician. There is also a prescription formulation combining benzoyl peroxide with the antibiotic erythromycin.

Topical Retinoids

How does Retin-A help acne?

Retin-A is the brand name for vitamin A acid, or tretinoin, a topical prescription treatment for acne that has recently received wide publicity as a treatment for wrinkles.

As discussed in the second question and answer of this chapter acne develops when the follicle becomes plugged. Tretinoin breaks up the waxy plug. When tretinoin was introduced over 15 years ago, it was considered a major breakthrough in acne therapy.

Tretinoin is especially useful for noninflammatory acne that consists primarily of comedones (blackheads and whiteheads), but it is also effective in treating inflammatory acne since inflammatory lesions start as microcomedones.

The skin may become red and peel when tretinoin therapy is initiated, but after a few weeks the skin adapts to the irritation and begins to look better. Irritation is most apt to occur in those with fair or sensitive skin. In addition, it is not uncommon for tretinoin to trigger a flareup of acne at the beginning of the treatment. Tretinoin also increases sensitivity to the sun, so it's necessary for those taking the drug to wear a sunblock whenever in the sun.

Tretinoin comes in various forms—gels, creams, and solutions—and in various concentrations. Your dermatologist may vary the form and concentration and frequency of application to minimize irritation.

Another retinoid, isotretinoin, has shown promising results when applied topically for the treatment of both noninflammatory and inflammatory acne. It had not yet been approved by the FDA for topical use at the time of this writing.

Oral Retinoids for Severe Acne

I've heard about Accutane®, but doesn't it have serious side effects? Please provide all pertinent information.

Accutane (isotretinoin) is an oral drug that is a derivative of vitamin A. Dermatologists consider Accutane to be the most important advance made in recent years in the treatment of severe acne that resists other kinds of therapy. It enables dermatologists, for the first time, to successfully treat the most severe cases of cystic acne that cause scarring.

Isotretinoin has an effect on all the processes that produce acne: It suppresses the activity of the sebaceous glands, reduces the bacterial population in the sebaceous follicles, and normalizes the abnormal process of keratinization in the follicle; it also has anti-inflammatory effects.

Acne may start to clear as early as the end of the first month of Accutane therapy and continue to improve throughout the treatment period, which is usually four to five months long. (Some patients may not see improvement for several months, however, and some may get even worse before they get better.) Not only is there great improvement, but it usually lasts for many months, or even years. Generally, after a year or two, oiliness returns and some superficial acne lesions may recur. A second course of treatment can be prescribed if necessary, but only a few cases require retreatment.

Unfortunately, isotretinoin has many side effects and must be administered under close medical supervision. The most serious side effect is that it produces serious birth defects in a high percentage of children born of mothers who take this drug during early pregnancy. Thus, it must not be used under any circumstances by women who are pregnant, and all women of childbearing potential must use adequate contraceptive procedures for one month before therapy, throughout therapy, and for one month after therapy. This problem is discussed further in the following question and answer.

Since isotretinoin suppresses production of sebum, the skin may become excessively dry and itchy. The lips may become severely chapped and inflamed. Other side effects include nosebleeds, sore gums, dry eyes (which may interfere with the wearing of contact lenses), other eye problems including night blindness, muscle aches and pains, changes in the bones and nervous system, hair loss, and abnormalities in the body's blood lipids (fats).

There also may be increased sensitivity to the sun. It appears that most, if not all, of these changes are reversible once therapy is stopped.

Before the drug is administered, certain laboratory tests must be performed on the patient's blood. If the findings are normal and the patient has no contraindications on physical examination and understands the nature of the treatment and the side effects, the drug can be taken. During therapy, blood tests may need to be performed every two to four weeks. Continuation of therapy depends on the results of the laboratory tests as well as the patient's response to the drug.

Accutane and Birth Defects

Please provide details about possible birth defects that may occur from taking Accutane.

Accutane (isotretinoin) is a potent drug that provides significant benefits for severe, cystic, nodular cases of acne that have not responded to other forms of therapy, as discussed in the previous answer.

The potential of Accutane to produce severe birth defects is the most serious side effect associated with its use. The drug is what is called a potent teratogenic agent. The effect on the fetus occurs very early in pregnancy (as early as two to four weeks), at a time when a woman does not know she is pregnant.

Accutane must not be used under any circumstances by women who are pregnant or actively trying to become pregnant. *A woman absolutely must not become pregnant while taking the drug, or for one month after therapy is stopped.* Before a dermatologist will prescribe isotretinoin for any female of childbearing age, the patient must have used an excellent, effective contraceptive technique for at least one month since her last normal menstrual period. The contraceptive technique must be continued throughout therapy and for one month after the drug is stopped. If the patient (or the physician) does not understand what constitutes effective contraception, she should have gynecological counseling. She must also have a reliable, sensitive blood pregnancy test done within two weeks of initiating therapy to ensure that she is not pregnant. It is advisable to do pregnancy tests monthly during therapy.

After therapy is stopped and the drug has cleared the body (it takes one month), a woman can safely become pregnant. Future children will not be affected. An analogy can be made to German measles during pregnancy: While the fetus may be affected, subsequent pregnancies will not be.

With the cooperation of the manufacturers, an extensive physician and patient education and awareness program has been developed that your dermatologist is likely to use if you are a woman of childbearing potential.

The drug has no effect on sperm, so a man can safely take the drug without any fear that a child he may father while on the drug will have birth defects.

Sulfur, Resorcin, and Salicylic Acid in Acne Medications

How beneficial are topical acne treatment products that contain salicylic acid, resorcin, or sulfur?

These ingredients were used alone or in combination as the active ingredients in most nonprescription acne medications before the advent of benzoyl peroxide. They are less popular today, but still have a place in acne therapy.

Sulfur alone or in combination with resorcin is helpful in healing lesions. These agents also have some antibacterial effects and some effects on the cells lining the follicle. Products containing sulfur and resorcin may be tinted in flesh tones to help conceal blemishes.

Salicylic acid acts on the follicular cells, thereby helping to unblock plugged follicles, but it is not as potent as tretinoin. It can help to prevent new lesions because it affects the abnormal desquamation process. It is most beneficial for mild cases of acne with a lot of small blackheads.

Intralesional Injections of Corticosteroids

How does injecting acne lesions with steroids help?

This is one of the techniques that dermatologists utilize for the improvement of nodulocystic lesions. The corticosteroids are anti-inflammatory, and when they are injected into inflamed nodulocystic lesions the cysts shrink very quickly. The sooner a cyst is injected the better, as the longer a cyst exists, the more likely it is to produce scarring. The injection of corticosteroids is not effective if there is no inflammation.

Cryosurgery

My dermatologist gave me a dry ice treatment for my acne last week. What does this do?

This treatment is referred to as cryosurgery because it involves light freezing of the skin. One form of cryosurgery used for acne utilizes carbon dioxide (dry ice) slush made by grinding up solid dry ice and mixing it with acetone. Sometimes sulfur is added to the slush. Liquid nitrogen and solid dry ice are also used for cryosurgery.

Cryosurgery may help reduce inflammation. It can be effective in minimizing (but not removing) acne scars.

If you have questions about the treatments your dermatologist is providing, you should discuss them. It is important that you understand the therapy being used for your acne, and for you and your dermatologist to work together to achieve the best results.

Cleansing and Acne

Should I wash my face more often if I have acne? Is it necessary to use a special soap?

Dermatologists generally recommend washing the face two or three times a day to remove the excess oil, bacteria, and dead cells from the skin surface. But washing must be done gently; overwashing can actually aggravate acne.

It is generally not necessary to use a special soap unless your dermatologist recommends that you do so. Medicated and abrasive soaps may, in fact, cause too much dryness because topical acne medications also produce drying and peeling.

Abrasives

Is it beneficial to use abrasives such as complexion brushes or abrasive sponges for cleansing when you have acne?

Abrasive cleansers produce mild irritation and peeling, which are supposed to help unclog plugged pores. While they may be of some benefit when used properly, the tendency is to use them too frequently or too vigorously, resulting in red, irritated skin that is overly dry. Some dermatologists believe that abrasives do not provide any special benefits and are too irritating for most people, and that they may actually aggravate acne. People with fair, sensitive skin must be especially careful when using abrasives as the skin is more easily irritated.

Zinc

Will taking zinc tablets help my acne?

Oral zinc was reported in recent years to aid in the treatment of acne. However, it is generally accepted by dermatologists that zinc has no specific value in the treatment of acne. Many better treatments are available.

Hormones and Acne

Is acne related to any hormonal imbalance? Will hormones help acne? I heard that birth control pills are effective.

The activity of the sebaceous (oil) glands is regulated by male hormones (androgens), in both men and women. Very few individuals with acne have any hormonal imbalances. Development of the sebaceous glands is essential for acne to occur. However, under certain circumstances, particularly in women, endocrinological abnormalities may play a role in acne. In most of these cases, the women have ongoing acne that does not respond well to the various therapeutic approaches. Furthermore, there are a few severe endocrinological disorders that have acne as part of their clinical spectrum.

If hormonal therapy is indicated, estrogens (female hormones) are usually administered to suppress sebaceous gland activity. In the past, oral contraceptives containing high dosages of estrogens were utilized. Today, however, there is a trend toward the use of oral contraceptives containing lower doses of estrogen. Some of these may be less effective than others, and a dermatologist should be consulted. Sometimes oral contraceptives are used in combination with corticosteroids to inhibit the adrenal glands, which may also produce androgens. However, as stated earlier, the number of women who require hormonal therapy to control acne is relatively small. If you suspect a hormonal abnormality, you should consult your gynecologist and/or dermatologist.

Shaving and Acne

Shaving is uncomfortable because of my acne. Which method is best? Any tips would be welcomed.

No one method of shaving is best for patients with acne. Some men find blade shaving more comfortable, while others prefer electric shavers. Sometimes it's more comfortable to rotate between the two. A few individuals must stop shaving altogether, at least temporarily.

If you are using a wet-shaving technique, be sure to adequately soften the beard by soaking the beard with warm water and shaving lather for at least a minute or two before you start to shave. It may be more comfortable to shave with the grain. Allow enough time to shave lightly and carefully. Try to avoid daily shaving.

Additional information on shaving is found in Chapter 10.

What to Do About Blackheads

I am plagued by blackheads in spite of frequent cleansing. What do you recommend?

Blackheads have nothing to do with dirt, as explained in the discussion of common myths elsewhere in this chapter. Blackheads and whiteheads are the initial lesions of acne and therefore must be treated properly.

Over-the-counter products containing ingredients such as salicylic acid are sometimes helpful for removing blackheads. You must be careful, however, to avoid excessive dryness and irritation. Read and follow the manufacturer's directions for use. If the skin becomes too dry or irritated, use the product less often.

Wash the face twice a day with a mild cleanser to remove excess oil. But be careful not to wash too much or too vigorously or you will irritate the skin. For the same reason, be cautious about using abrasive cleansers.

Avoid oily, greasy cosmetics. Wear oil-free or water-based products that are labeled noncomedogenic or nonacnegenic.

If these measures don't work, see your dermatologist, who can prescribe more potent treatments such as topical tretinoin.

Don't squeeze blackheads! You may injure the follicular wall and cause the contents of the comedo to break through the wall of the follicle into the surrounding tissue, where it will produce inflammation. Your dermatologist can either extract the blackheads or show you the proper technique for removing them yourself.

Hyperpigmentation from Acne

As my acne blemishes heal, they leave dark spots on the skin. What can I do about this? The spots are almost as unattractive as the acne.

Irritation and injury to the skin from acne can stimulate the pigment-forming cells in the area to overproduce, leaving dark spots when the acne lesions heal. This reaction is referred to as postinflammatory hyperpigmentation. It is more apt to appear in individuals with darker complexions and can be a special problem for blacks. It can also be more of a problem in people who pick at their acne.

The hyperpigmentation will gradually fade over the course of several to many months. You can conceal the hyperpigmentation with a masking cosmetic.

Acne from Cosmetics

Is it true that some cosmetics cause acne? If so, which products should I avoid?

Cosmetics can cause two different types of acne. One type consists primarily of comedones (whiteheads and blackheads) and usually occurs after a product has been used for several months. The production of comedones is referred to as comedogenic activity. The other type of reaction consists of the development of inflammatory lesions (pustules) and occurs more rapidly, usually within a week or two of using a new cosmetic or regimen of cosmetics. This action is referred to as pustulogenic or acnegenic action.

Certain ingredients incorporated into cosmetics, especially creamy makeups and moisturizers, have been reported to be either comedogenic or acnegenic, or both, when tested as individual ingredients. As a natural extension of this, lists of such ingredients have appeared in both medical and consumer articles, prompting both physicians and patients to carefully read the ingredient listings on cosmetic packages. However, in actual use, some products free of any of these ingredients produce reactions while some products that contain offending ingredients do not produce reactions. The consensus of opinion now is that the final product, not individual ingredients, must determine whether products are comedogenic or acnegenic.

Tests have been developed that can fairly accurately predict whether a product will be comedogenic or acnegenic in actual use. Manufacturers have been urged to carry out testing to determine if their products are noncomedogenic or nonacnegenic and to label the products accordingly.

If you have experienced comedogenic or acnegenic reactions from cosmetics, you should look for products that are labeled as noncomedogenic or nonacnegenic. You are less likely to experience a reaction from using one of these products. If you continue to have reactions, consult a dermatologist.

Friction and Acne (Acne Mechanica)

My dermatologist told me not to sit with my chin in my hands as this will aggravate my acne. Why?

Sitting with your chin in your hand may lead to unconscious manipulation of your face, which can aggravate acne as much as deliberate squeezing. It may also cause mechanical irritation, which worsens acne. This is sometimes called acne mechanica.

Mechanical irritation may also be caused by clothing, for instance, headbands, football pads, and other occlusive or rough clothing. The mechanical irritation is usually complicated by accompanying conditions of heat and humidity.

Another variation on the theme of acne mechanica occurs when individuals scrub their skin too often and too vigorously with harsh, irritating cleansers or abrasives in the mistaken belief that such vigorous cleansing will rid the skin of acne.

Acne and Heredity

I had severe acne as a teenager. Does this mean my children will also have acne?

The exact role of heredity in acne is not clearly understood. We do know that people with severe acne are more likely to have children with acne; however, a parent with acne should not be concerned that his child will necessarily develop it as well.

One of the problems in determining the role of heredity in acne is the fact that acne is so common. Acne affects about 85% of the population at some time.

Acne and the Environment

Why does my acne seem to get worse in hot, humid weather?

In sections of the country where the humidity may vary greatly, acne may flare up during prolonged hot, humid spells. The mechanism has not been clearly established. It is sometimes referred to as "tropical acne." This reaction is fairly abrupt, occurring within a day or two of the change in environment. Consult your dermatologist about how to deal with this problem.

Acne in Adult Women

Why have I developed acne at the age of 26 when I never had it as a teenager?

Acne most often occurs during or soon after puberty and diminishes in the late teens or early twenties, but it may persist in some individuals for many years.

However, there are some women like you in whom acne does not appear until the twenties, or even the thirties. We do not know why this happens. While the stresses of modern life, such as competing in the workplace, have been mentioned as potential causes, there is no good evidence that this is so. Cosmetics have also been blamed, as discussed in a separate question and answer in this chapter. In some cases there may be hormonal imbalances, also described in this chapter.

You should consult a dermatologist for treatment.

Sex, Dirt, Diet and Other Myths

Is it true that sexual activity will make acne worse? If I wash my face frequently enough, will the acne go away? What diet should I follow?

There are many myths associated with acne and three of the most common are: 1) acne is caused by dirt, so frequent cleansing will prevent or cure it; 2) sexual activity causes acne or makes it worse; and 3) eating the wrong foods causes acne. None of these has any basis in fact.

Acne is not caused by dirt. You can have the cleanest skin in the world and still develop acne, or you can have a filthy face and never have a blemish. Children before puberty do not develop acne no matter how dirty they are. Washing the face too often, especially with harsh, medicated, or abrasive cleansers, may actually make acne worse.

There is no relationship between acne and sexual activity. However, male sex hormones must be circulating in the body for acne to occur since androgenic hormones stimulate the sebaceous glands. Prepubertal children and eunuchs don't develop acne.

Diet does not have any significant effect on acne, and following the strictest diet will not prevent or improve it. There is no evidence that foods such as chocolate, potato chips, or other greasy foods, and dairy products (which teenagers usually enjoy) cause or aggravate acne. For example, eating greasy foods does not affect the skin's oiliness (which is due to the oil secreted by the skin's sebaceous glands). The only time milk must be avoided is when you are taking tetracycline for acne and then just for one to 1½ hours before and two hours after. The only foods that dermatologists may sometimes recommend that acne patients avoid are foods with a high iodine content, such as shellfish, because excessive amounts of iodine may cause flareups of existing acne. However, iodine should not be avoided altogether or a goiter may develop. Generally, dermatologists simply recommend that acne patients have a well-balanced diet. However, if your acne gets worse when you eat a specific food, it is best to avoid that food.

Lithium and Acne

I am taking lithium. Can it cause acne?

Many of those who take lithium develop acne, usually consisting of comedones and worse on the face. The mechanism is unknown. Treatment is the same as for ordinary acne. It should be remembered, however, that lithium can interact with oral tetracycline, a drug used to treat ordinary inflammatory acne.

Chloracne

What is chloracne?

Chloracne refers to a type of acne originally due to chlorinated compounds found in industry. Chloracne is most commonly a reaction to cutting oils, but coal tar derivatives, chlorinated hydrocarbons, and dioxin compounds have also been implicated.

Chloracne is not confined to the face; in fact, it is more common on areas where contaminated clothing comes into contact with the skin. The lesions are usually highly inflammatory, with large nodules and cysts. There are also giant comedones.

Tar and Acne

I work with tar on my job and I heard it can cause acne. Is this true?

Those working with tar products may develop acne much as happens with chloracne (see previous answer). It has the same clinical spectrum, and the offending ingredient may be common to both products. However, it is more likely that the reaction to tars will be folliculitis rather than chloracne.

Newborn Acne

Is it possible for newborn infants to have acne?

Acne in the newborn occurs occasionally, usually on and near the nose. It is probably related to stimulation of the fetus' sebaceous glands by maternal hormones during pregnancy. The condition almost always clears spontaneously, but occasionally tiny pitted scars may be left. The appearance of newborn acne may indicate a greater risk of developing acne later in life.

Steroid (Corticosteroid) Acne

I've been taking steroids for a medical problem and have developed acne. Is there any relationship?

Acne frequently accompanies systemic corticosteroid treatment. It most often occurs with long-term treatment but may appear just a few weeks after starting the treatment. The acne lesions usually all look the same: small, dome-shaped papules one to three millimeters in diameter. Comedones may appear later. The shoulders, trunk, and face may be involved, The lesions remain until steroid treatment ends, and the skin then gradually returns to normal. Conventional acne treatment is helpful in controlling steroid acne.

Collagen Injections for Acne Scars

Will collagen injections remove my acne scars? Are the results permanent?

You must accept the fact that there is no currently available technique that will completely remove acne scars, especially the deep, pitted scars that follow severe acne.

Collagen injection is one of the newer techniques that can improve some scars, especially if they are shallow and crater-like. A purified form of liquid bovine collagen suspended in salt water is injected under the scar to elevate it. The site must be overcorrected initially so that when the salt water is absorbed into the body, enough collagen remains to raise the scar. The total number of injections needed depends on the size and location of scars.

The treatment site looks bruised, discolored, and swollen for two or three days and then generally returns to normal. However, a few people experience bumps that persist for weeks. Some people (about 4%) may be allergic to the collagen, so a skin test is necessary before the first injection is given. A few other people (about 1%) will become allergic to collagen after treatment begins. Anyone with a history of autoimmune diseases cannot have collagen injections.

Finally, the results from collagen injections are not permanent. Within six months to two years, depending on the type of collagen used, the collagen will be absorbed and treatments must be repeated.

Dermabrasion for Acne Scars

How effective is dermabrasion for removing acne scars? What does it involve?

Dermabrasion (skin planing) is one of the techniques that may be used to improve the appearance of acne scarring. Unfortunately, no method currently exists that will completely erase the pits and scars that may remain after acne. What you can do is make the scars less obvious. Makeup may also cover the area more smoothly after dermabrasion.

Dermabrasion involves removal of the outer layers of skin. The facial skin is anesthetized and frozen sequentially in small sections. Freezing stiffens the skin so it is firm for abrading. Then a rapidly rotating wire brush, diamond fraise, or serrated wheel is stroked across the skin to plane or smooth it, much as wood is planed or sanded smooth.

There may be considerable swelling for a day or two following dermabrasion. Crusts, which will come off in 10–20 days, cover the operation sites. The new skin that forms is smooth, but it is likely to remain red for two to six months. The skin is thin and therefore more sensitive to sunlight, so overexposure to the sun must be avoided for several months.

Dermabrasion does not improve the appearance of all types of scars. It works best on shallow, broader scars rather than deeply pitted "icepick" scars. The degree of improvement will usually range from 20 to 70%; it is never 100%. Fair-complexioned individuals are better candidates (in dark-complexioned individuals, the pigmentation is often irregular because of pigment cell damage). For this reason, the treatment is not recommended for blacks. Also, blacks have a greater risk of keloid formation after dermabrasion.

Dermabrasion produces few complications as long as it is done by a physician experienced in the technique, such as a dermatological surgeon. Patients must be carefully selected to help prevent dissatisfaction with the results achieved. Many dermatologists are not very enthusiastic about dermabrasion because the results may be less than the patient expects. Dermabrasion can be repeated to improve the results, but each planing provides proportionally less improvement.

Treatment of Deep "Icepick" Scars

Can anything be done for deep, pitted, icepick-type acne scars?

Unfortunately, these are the most difficult acne scars to treat. Procedures such as dermabrasion and collagen injections are of limited benefit. More improvement may be obtained by either punch excision, punch-graft excision, or punch elevation, but you must realize that no technique will leave you with a smooth skin.

In punch excision, the scar is removed with a small punch-type instrument and the wound is then stitched together with fine sutures. In punch-graft excision, the icepick scar is excised with a skin punch and a punch graft from another site (usually behind the ear) is placed and sutured in the excision site. The third technique, punch-graft elevation, also involves removal of a plug with the pitted scar tissue, but instead of replacing it with a plug of skin from another site, the plug of scar tissue is replaced, in an elevated position. After healing, the elevated area can be smoothed down with electrosurgery. Small scars remain from each of these procedures, but the scars are less obvious than before. Also, they provide a better surface for the application of cosmetics.

Your dermatologist can advise you about whether you are a suitable candidate for treatment.

23

Psoriasis

Psoriasis Is Not Contagious

A friend of mine has developed psoriasis. Other friends are afraid they will catch it from her. Is this possible? Any information will be welcomed.

Psoriasis (*so-RYE-uh-sis*) is a chronic skin disease that affects about three million people in the United States. The cause is unknown but we do know that it *is not* contagious.

Psoriasis results from an overproduction of skin cells in the epidermis, the outer layer of skin. Normally it takes about a month for the cells of the epidermis to mature and be shed from the surface. In psoriasis this maturation occurs in a week or less. Lesions of psoriasis appear as red patches covered with thick, silvery scales. Psoriasis may be limited to a small area or cover large portions of the body. The scalp, elbows, knees, arms, and legs are the most commonly affected sites. The nails may also be deformed.

Psoriasis occurs in both men and women with equal frequency and may begin at any age. It is often first diagnosed during the teenage years or early adulthood. Heredity seems to play a role since many patients with psoriasis have other family members with the disease.

Many things may aggravate psoriasis or cause flare-ups. Patches of psoriasis may develop at sites of such minor injuries as cuts, scratches, minor abrasions, and severe sunburn. Psoriasis can also be triggered by infections—for example, strep throat—and by certain drugs, including lithium, propranolol, and chloroquine. Emotional stress can make psoriasis worse.

People who live in cold-weather climates frequently have flare-ups of psoriasis in winter when they are unable to benefit from moderate exposure to sunlight, which usually helps control psoriasis.

Your friend must understand that she has a chronic disease (like diabetes or arthritis) that has a tendency to flare up and then subside. However, in most cases, remission can be obtained with proper therapy. Your friend should be under the care of a dermatologist, who can tailor treatment to her individual case; no one form of therapy is ideal for everyone. Many advances have been made in the treatment of psoriasis, and the dermatologist should be able to keep her disease under adequate control if she faithfully follows the prescribed treatment regimen. Your friend can obtain more information on psoriasis by writing to the American Academy of Dermatology.

Different Forms of Psoriasis

Are there different kinds of psoriasis?

Yes. The lesions of psoriasis differ in their clinical appearance, duration, and location.

The most common form starts out with red, flat, scaly lesions. The scales are usually silver. The top scales flake off easily and frequently, somewhat like a piece of mica, while those below stick to the underlying skin, so when they are removed, bleeding occurs. The lesions may grow to cover large areas.

The elbows, knees, arms, legs, and scalp are most commonly involved. The lesions are frequently symmetrical on both sides of the body.

Psoriasis also commonly affects the nails. The signs of nail psoriasis include pitting, separation of the nail from the nail bed, and thickening or crumbling of the nail plate. Psoriasis of the nail is difficult to treat.

Another type of psoriasis is called inverse psoriasis because it involves the folds of the skin in the armpit, under the breast, in the groin area, in the cleft between the buttocks, and around the genitals.

Guttate (droplike) psoriasis occurs primarily in children and young adults. Many small, red, droplike, scaly spots appear all over the trunk, limbs, and scalp. This variety of psoriasis is often preceded by a sore throat caused by streptococcal or viral organisms. It often clears up spontaneously after four weeks or more and is the least likely form to become chronic.

A very severe, uncommon form, pustular psoriasis, often requires hospitalization and vigorous therapy.

About 5% of psoriasis patients have arthritis. Some of them have specific rheumatic diseases unrelated to the psoriasis, but others have psoriatic arthritis with joint deformities. The acute symptoms of arthritis associated with psoriasis sometimes improve when the skin manifestations of the disease improve, but the joint deformities are usually permanent. Early treatment by your dermatologist is therefore important.

Current Therapy Can Help

What treatments are currently recommended for psoriasis? Can they really help? I have had psoriasis for years and have almost given up.

While psoriasis can't be cured, proper medical treatment can usually provide significant relief and sometimes even prolonged remission. Since psoriasis involves an accelerated production of skin cells, the main goal of treatment is to slow down this process.

Treatment must be individualized to take into account your overall medical condition, age, and lifestyle, and the severity and duration of psoriasis. Various treatments, one at a time or in combination, and visits to a dermatologist may be necessary before psoriasis is brought under control.

Prescription medications containing cortisone, salicylic acid, tar, or anthralin may be recommended alone or in combination with natural sunlight or special ultraviolet sunlamps. Sunlight exposure helps about 95% of people who can tan easily but must be used cautiously by people who sunburn easily.

The most severe forms of psoriasis may require oral medications with or without combined ultraviolet light treatments. PUVA therapy, which involves the use of psoralen drugs plus ultraviolet light, is discussed in detail later in this chapter. Treatment with the drug etretinate is also discussed. Methotrexate, a form of chemotherapy, can also be given in recalcitrant cases.These medications may have significant side effects and require a dermatologist's close supervision.

Bland moisturizing creams and lotions can help to relieve the itching and dryness, thus improving the patient's appearance and making him or her more comfortable.

There is no reason for anyone today to suffer the "heartbreak of psoriasis." Most patients can be helped by treatment, but control entails periodic visits to a dermatologist and careful adherence to the treatments prescribed.

Psoriasis Can't Be Cured

My psoriasis has completely disappeared. Does this mean it is cured?

Sorry, but the answer is no. There is no cure for psoriasis, although the disease does have a tendency to flare up and then subside. Sometimes treatment can cause psoriasis to go into remission for many months or even years, but it may flare up again at any time.

Dermatologists point out that one of the problems in treating psoriasis is that when patients obtain temporary control or clearing of the disease, they stop using their medication. Then psoriasis may flare up again. Don't be fooled. Keep up the treatment regimen and office-visit schedule your dermatologist has prescribed, and your psoriasis just might stay in remission for quite a while.

Scalp Psoriasis

I have severe psoriasis of the scalp. What treatment is recommended?

The scalp is a frequent site for psoriasis. Often it is mistaken for severe dandruff, seborrheic dermatitis, or eczema.

The treatment for psoriasis of the scalp depends on the severity of the disease. A wide variety of over-the-counter and prescription shampoos, oils, solutions, and sprays are available. Many of them contain coal tar (see the following question and answer). Certain treatments are not very cosmetically elegant, so some patients may not be willing to use them. Medicated shampoos should be left on the scalp for several minutes before being rinsed out.

To prevent dryness of the hair, conditioners can be used after shampooing.

Coal Tar Therapy

Is coal tar therapy for psoriasis safe? I've read that coal tar causes cancer.

Coal tar has been used for more than 100 years to treat psoriasis. Improvements in manufacturing have produced coal tar products that smell better and are not messy. Higher-concentration prescriptions can be compounded for difficult cases. Treatment regimens may include daily coal tar baths, in some cases followed by application of various topical preparations. Coal tar is the active ingredient in many medicated shampoos.

While crude coal tar is known to induce cancer under certain conditions, the federal government has approved its continued use in topical dermatological preparations. Coal tar in conjunction with ultraviolet light (the Goeckerman regimen) has been used since the 1920s as routine therapy for psoriasis. No increase in skin cancer has been detected in patients treated with the Goeckkerman regimen.

PUVA for Psoriasis

What is PUVA therapy for psoriasis? Do I have to go to a doctor for the treatment?

PUVA therapy is a relatively new treatment for psoriasis that must be administered under the supervision of a dermatologist. Patients are given a drug called psoralen prior to being exposed to an accurately measured amount of a special type of ultraviolet light (UVA), thus the name PUVA (psoralen plus UVA light).

This treatment is one of the forms of therapy used in patients who have failed to respond to other treatments or who have psoriasis over more than 30% of their body. It is effective in 85 to 90% of patients.

PUVA must be administered by your dermatologist because the amount of drug as well as the ultraviolet-A light therapy must be carefully monitored. A severe sunburn may result from over treatment. In the average case, about 25 treatments are given over a two- or three-month span. Then the patient usually requires maintenance therapy at a reduced treatment frequency. Relapses can occur.

Because the drug can remain in the lens of the eye, a patient being treated with PUVA must wear a special type of dark glasses after taking the drug, during therapy, and during daylight for 24 hours after the light treatment to prevent damage to the eyes.

Chronic photochemotherapy with PUVA increases a person's risk of skin aging, freckling, and possibly skin cancer. Those who should not be considered candidates for this treatment modality are patients below the age of 18, pregnant women, people who have had previous exposure to arsenic or x-ray radiation, and people with skin cancer, severe eye disease, or diseases such as lupus erythematosus that are aggravated by ultraviolet therapy.

Etretinate for Psoriasis

I've heard about a new treatment for psoriasis that utilizes something called a retinoid. Can you tell me anything about this treatment? Could it help my severe psoriasis?

A retinoid is a chemical that is a close derivative of vitamin A. One retinoid, etretinate (Tegison®), given orally, has been proven to be effective in treating certain cases of psoriasis. Another retinoid, called 13-cis-retinoic acid or isotretinoin (Accutane®), given orally, has been proven to be very successful in the management of acne (see the discussion of acne treatments in Chapter 22). Retinoids must be prescribed by a physician.

Etretinate is a potent drug that is used to treat only severe or disabling cases of psoriasis that do not respond to other forms of therapy. Most patients experience side effects, some of which are serious. Because etretinate can produce severe birth defects, women of childbearing age must not be pregnant when they first start the drug or become pregnant while they are taking it. They must have a negative, reliable pregnancy test before starting therapy and begin medication on the second day of the next menstrual period. Women also must use an effective contraceptive during the administration of etretinate, and, since the drug is excreted slowly from the body, contraception must be continued for *at least* two years after the drug is stopped. The harmful effects on the fetus are most likely to occur very early in pregnancy. It is critical, therefore, to be certain that a woman is using effective contraception while taking the drug, as its effect on the fetus may occur before a woman is aware of her pregnancy.

Side effects that involve the skin and mucous membranes include: peeling of the palms, soles, and fingertips, itching, dry skin, hair loss, chapped lips, dry nose, and dry eyes, making it necessary for those wearing contact lens to use artificial tears. These symptoms disappear when the drug is stopped.

Other adverse reactions include bone and joint pain and headaches. There are many other side effects, which your dermatologist will explain to you. In addition, patients taking etretinate require frequent laboratory monitoring.

Despite these problems, etretinate can provide considerable improvement for patients whose psoriasis has not responded to other forms of therapy.

If you have severe psoriasis, you should be under the care of a dermatologist. It is most likely that you can be helped by one or more of the various treatments that are now available. Your dermatologist will help you select the most appropriate treatment for your condition.

24

Herpes Infections

Different Types of Herpes Infections

What causes herpes infections? Are there different types of herpes infections?

There are some 50 related herpes viruses. They include those responsible for fever blisters (herpes simplex), infectious mononucleosis (Epstein-Barr virus), chicken pox (varicella), and shingles (herpes zoster).

Questions about specific herpes infections are answered in the remainder of this chapter.

Fever Blisters and Cold Sores

I am plagued by recurrent fever blisters. Is there any difference between herpes infections on the face and genital herpes?

There are two types of herpes simplex virus (HSV): Type 1 and Type 2. Studies show that most people contract Type 1, which most often affects the lips, mouth, nose, chin, or cheeks, but may also affect the genital area. Type 2 usually occurs in the genital area following sexual contact with an infected person. (See the following question and answer for a detailed discussion of Type 2 and genital herpes.)

HSV Type 1 is usually responsible for the sores commonly

referred to as fever blisters or cold sores. While the initial (primary) infection may occur in adulthood, it most commonly occurs during childhood from close contact with family members or friends who carry the virus and transmit it to the child by kissing or other close personal contact. In the initial infection, the symptoms, if any, may be barely noticeable. However, in a small number of cases, the initial infection may be very severe, even requiring hospitalization.

The first symptoms of an HSV infection may be itching, tingling, and/or red, sensitive skin. Then tiny, fluid-filled blisters appear, with the number varying from one to a whole cluster. The blisters generally break spontaneously or as a result of minor trauma, allowing the fluid contents to ooze out. Eventually scabs form. When these fall off, the skin is usually slightly red. The whole process usually takes one to two weeks.

Although primary infections heal completely, rarely leaving a scar, the virus remains in the body, migrating to nerve cells where it remains in an inactive state. Most people will not experience another infection or recurrence. Others, like you, will be plagued with recurrences, either in the same location as the first infection or nearby. The infections may recur every few weeks or only infrequently.

Colds, fever, exposure to the sun, and the onset of a menstrual period may trigger recurrent infections. However, for many individuals the recurrences are unpredictable and have no recognizable precipitating cause. The recurrent infections are usually mild and self-limited.

The clinical appearance of an HSV infection is often so characteristic that both the physician and the patient can diagnose it by just looking at the lesions. If the diagnosis is uncertain, however, it may be confirmed by examining scrapings from the base of the lesion, or by doing a virus culture.

While there are many over-the-counter treatments promoted for treating fever blisters, in general they are not very effective. Therefore, if you are plagued with recurrent herpes infections, you should consult a dermatologist. There is no vaccine to protect an individual from herpes infections; however, a prescription drug is now available that, if taken regularly, may shorten the duration of active infections and prevent recurrences.

Do not ever touch a herpes lesion and then touch the eye. Herpes infections around the eye may be quite serious, leading to inflammation and blindness. If you should develop a herpes infection around the eye, consult an ophthalmologist promptly.

Genital Herpes

I guess I am one of millions of people afflicted with genital herpes. Please provide complete information on the cause and treatment of this problem. Is it contracted only through sexual exposure?

Genital herpes infections are most often caused by herpes simplex virus (HSV) Type 2 and usually occur after sexual contact with an infected person. But sometimes genital herpes infections are caused by Type 1 HSV. This usually occurs through oral sexual exposure with someone who has a Type 1 infection on the face or mouth.

You certainly aren't alone if you have genital herpes. Experts agree that genital herpes has reached epidemic proportions, affecting anywhere between five and 20 million persons in the United States, or up to 20% of all sexually active adults. It has become one of the most common sexually transmitted diseases.

Lesions of herpes simplex virus Type 2 are usually found on the buttocks, penis, vagina, or cervix. They occur two to 20 days after contact with an infected person. While sexual intercourse is the most frequent means of transmission, infection may occur in the absence of any sexual contact.

The lesions may be accompanied by generalized symptoms such as fever and achy muscles. If the blisters are near the tip of the penis or in the vagina, there may be pain and burning on urination. Sexual intercourse may also be painful. Swollen and tender lymph glands in the groin are common.

After the initial attack, the virus moves to nerve cells near the spinal cord, remaining there until provoked by a trigger such as a menstrual period, fever, physical contact, or stress.

Both primary and recurrent infections may be preceded by pain or unusual tenderness at the site where the lesions will develop. Pain sensation is not transmitted from the cervix, so a small number of women with infections involving the cervix may not even be aware that they have an infection.

Compresses, sitz baths, local anesthetics, and oral anti-inflammatory medications can help to relieve discomfort if a recurrence occurs. In the past there was no specific treatment for herpes infections. Now, however, there is a prescription antiviral drug that can shorten the course of the disease if given early in an acute attack. The drug also may prevent recurrences while it is being taken. You should see your dermatologist for further advice.

Herpes is very contagious; between 200,000 and 500,000 persons, from all socioeconomic classes and ethnic groups, "catch" genital herpes each year.

If tingling, burning, itching, or tenderness—signs of a recurrence—are present in an area of the body where you have had a previous herpes infection, it is important to abstain from sexual relations or oral-genital contact in order to prevent potential spread to other individuals. If abstinence is not observed, a rubber condom should be used, as the virus cannot penetrate rubber. Towels and clothing should not be shared.

Sexual Exposure and Genital Herpes

Must a person abstain from sexual activity during an outbreak of genital herpes?

If one has an active genital herpes simplex infection and sexual activity is not stopped, you should initiate measures to protect your sexual partner. If no precautions are taken, there is a very high risk of infecting your partner. Rubber condoms will help prevent the passage of the herpes simplex virus, but they will protect only the skin that is covered by the condom. Also, the condom must remain intact to be effective.

If no active or open lesions are present, spread of the disease is most unlikely. This is true even though virus particles may be shed for up to 18 days after healing has occurred. However, remember that lesions in the vagina or involving the cervix, or very small lesions, may be silent (asymptomatic).

Herpes Infections in Babies

Is it true that it is dangerous for an infant to be delivered vaginally if the mother has genital herpes? I heard that the baby may suffer brain damage.

A pregnant woman who has genital herpes at the time of delivery may transmit the virus to her baby as it passes through the birth canal. While it is estimated that only half of the infants delivered through an infected vagina acquire the disease, those who do may develop a severe, widespread infection. The baby can die or suffer severe damage, particularly mental retardation. Women who know that they have had genital herpes or who think they might have genital herpes during their pregnancy should tell their physicians so that preventive measures can be taken. A caesarean section is indicated for some patients.

Near the time of delivery, it is recommended that women with genital sores as well as those with a prior history of genital herpes be examined and tested for vaginal herpes. A diagnosis, in most instances, can be made in a few days by examining vaginal or cervical scrapings with a viral culture and PAP smear. The final decision on how to deliver the child is based on the relative risks for both the mother and the child.

Infants must also be protected from exposure to individuals who have active herpes infections on the skin. Therefore, family members, nursing staff, and friends with active HSV should not handle a newborn infant.

Pregnant women should avoid sexual contact, especially late in pregnancy, with a partner who has active genital herpes. The risk of vaginal infections from oral lesions in oral-genital sexual exposure should be recognized.

No special precautions need be taken by the woman who has inactive herpes (genital or nongenital) at term. When the mother's infection is not active, the infant is not at risk. However, you must remember that vaginal and cervical lesions may be asymptomatic.

Other Herpes Problems

Can herpes infections occur in areas other than the lips and genital areas?

Yes, and herpes simplex infections in different areas present special problems.

Infections on the fingers (common in physicians, dentists, and nurses) can be serious. Frequently they are disabling, recurring infections with associated lymphangitis, commonly known as blood poisoning: red streaks, chills, fever, pain, enlarged lymph glands. Herpes infections around the fingers are frequently misdiagnosed as streptococcal bacterial infections.

Herpes simplex infections of the eye are serious, painful, and disabling, and result in various degrees of eye damage. If there is any suggestion of a herpes infection of the eye, the patient should see an ophthalmologist as soon as possible for diagnosis and treatment.

Anal herpes simplex infections are most common in homosexuals. Significant discomfort is associated with defecation. Enlargement of the lymph glands in the groin may be present. Symptomatic treatment with sitz baths and local anesthetics helps, but a prescription antiviral drug that is now available is the treatment of choice. The presence of other venereal diseases should be excluded.

Herpes Zoster (Shingles)

What causes shingles? What treatments are recommended?

Herpes zoster (shingles) is a viral infection involving a nerve and the skin overlying the nerve. It is caused by the chicken pox virus and is not related to herpes simplex.

After a person has been infected with chicken pox, the virus may move to nerves and remain in an inactive state until some future time when it becomes activated and causes herpes zoster. This occurs in, at most, only 1–2% of those who have had chicken pox.

Shingles is characterized by the presence of small, grouped blisters that tend to follow the course of a nerve. The lesions involve only one side of the body. There is redness surrounding the blisters. Discomfort with itching, burning, increased skin sensitivity, and pain may occur before, during, or after the appearance of the lesions. The lesions usually last for two to four weeks. If severe or characterized by bleeding into the lesions, herpes zoster may result in scarring similar to that following a severe chicken pox infection. Sometimes even if there are few or no symptoms severe, long-lasting pain may occur, particularly in elderly patients. The duration and severity of the symptoms are unpredictable.

In many cases, the post-infection neuralgia is more distressing than the attack of shingles. Pain may persist for months or years. Treatment is often unsatisfactory.

Any nerve may be involved. The nerves involving the chest and body are most commonly affected. If the middle branch of the facial nerve is involved, there may be eye damage.

Shingles can be a serious problem, particularly in the elderly or those in whom immunity is naturally or specifically depressed. Prompt medical attention is indicated for all cases of shingles.

In the past, the treatment of shingles was primarily symptomatic, but a prescription antiviral drug used to treat herpes simplex has proven to be effective for many cases of shingles when administered in higher doses. However, the drug has not yet been approved for such treatment. A dermatologist may also prescribe various topical and oral drugs to treat the lesions and relieve pain. Antibiotics may be prescribed if the lesions become infected or are widespread and severe. Post-herpetic neuralgia may need constant care and even surgical approaches.

Chicken Pox

Does everyone get chicken pox during childhood? If my children catch it, what treatment is recommended? Will it leave scars?

Chicken pox is caused by the varicella virus, a member of the herpes family. A very small percentage of those with chicken pox may develop shingles (herpes zoster) later on in life.

Most people have chicken pox during childhood, but the disease may be mild, without a rash, and thus be mistaken by parents for a cold or the flu.

When an obvious case of chicken pox occurs, drying compresses may be used to speed healing and prevent secondary bacterial infection.

25

Nevi and Pigmentation Problems

Vitiligo

I have developed white patches of skin on my arms that my doctor says are patches of vitiligo. Please provide details about this disorder and any treatments that are available.

Vitiligo is a condition of unknown cause in which the major skin pigment, melanin, is not produced in certain areas of the skin. The irregularly shaped white patches of skin are most obvious and distressing for dark-skinned individuals, as the contrast between pigmented and nonpigmented skin is more noticeable.

Vitiligo may involve any portion of the skin. Common sites are exposed areas such as the face, neck, and hands; body folds such as armpits and groin; nipples; genitalia; and areas injured by cuts, scrapes, burns, etc.

Vitiligo affects at least 1% of the population. About half the people who develop vitiligo experience some pigment loss before the age of 20. Most people with the disorder are otherwise healthy.

There is no way to predict how much pigment an individual will lose. Vitiligo frequently begins with a rapid loss of pigment, which may be followed by a long period when the skin color does not change. Later the pigment loss may begin again. It is rare for anyone with vitiligo to regain full skin color spontaneously.

Treatment of vitiligo is not completely satisfactory. Two basic methods that might be tried by your dermatologist are attempting to restore the normal pigment (repigmentation) or removing the remaining pigment (depigmentation).

In repigmentation therapy, the patient is given a drug called psoralen and then exposed to controlled amounts of ultraviolet light—either natural sunlight or a sunlamp. The results of this type of therapy are variable.

The ideal candidate for repigmentation therapy is an individual whose pigment loss began within the last five years. In general, children and young adults respond better, but a candidate under 10 years old is unlikely to have the patience to stick with therapy. The treatment process is long and tedious. While most patients show some repigmentation, total repigmentation rarely occurs. The face responds best; hands rarely return to normal color.

If a person has vitiligo involving more than half of the body's exposed areas, he or she might be a candidate for depigmentation. A special depigmenting drug, called monobenzylether of hydroquinone, is applied to the skin to remove the remaining pigment. The drug must be carefully applied only to the area being depigmented. Some patients become allergic to this medication and therefore must discontinue therapy. Patients who achieve complete depigmentation are usually satisfied with the results. Of course, since the skin lacks pigment, it must be protected from the sun.

One of the best ways to deal with vitiligo may be to camouflage the depigmented areas so they are less obvious. Your dermatologist can provide information on special natural or synthetic stains that will color the depigmented areas and on masking cosmetics designed to cover birthmarks. The masking cosmetics may be of particular value on the face and neck.

Since the melanin pigment is the skin's most important natural protecting agent against sun damage, the areas of vitiligo must be protected from sun exposure. A sunblock with maximum protection (SPF 15 or greater) is a necessity. Or, in your case, since the vitiligo is on the arms, you can wear long sleeves to protect the depigmented areas from the sun.

For more information on vitiligo, you may want to contact the American Academy of Dermatology.

Hyperpigmentation of Black Skin

I am black, and every time I cut or injure my skin I'm left with dark spots. My friends have the same problem. What causes black skin to respond to injury in this way? Is there any way to prevent it?

Black skin has more melanin pigment and produces melanin more rapidly than white skin. Because of this difference, pigmentary disturbances are more apt to be seen in blacks than in whites.

The type of pigmentation problem you describe in which injured areas become darker than surrounding areas is called "post-inflammatory hyperpigmentation" because it usually occurs after an injury to the skin, such as a cut or an abrasion, or after a case of acne or other skin disorder.

The only way you can prevent post-inflammatory hyperpigmentation is to avoid the causative injury or skin problem, and this is usually impossible.

The hyperpigmented areas of skin usually fade in time. Bleaching preparations containing hydroquinone may be helpful in accelerating the return of your normal skin color. You must be careful, however, to apply the bleaching product only to the hyperpigmented areas as the product may also bleach out the normally pigmented skin, resulting in an even greater cosmetic defect.

Hyperpigmentation from Perfume

I've developed brown spots on my neck where I applied perfume before going to the beach. What caused this? Is it permanent?

Some perfumes contain ingredients called photosensitizers, which enhance the normal effect of sunlight on the skin. Thus, an individual may develop increased pigmentation (brown spots) on areas to which perfume has been applied before sun exposure. Oil of bergamot, an ingredient quite commonly found in perfumes, is such a photosensitizer. Aftershave and men's colognes may also contain such photosensitizers as plant extracts from limes. These

extracts contain psoralens, which are well-known photosensitizers.

This type of spotty pigmentation is known as "berlock" (or
"berlocque") dermatitis. While the reaction may be cosmetically
disturbing, it is not serious.

There is no effective treatment and the pigmentation generally
persists for quite a while. Your best bet is to camouflage the discoloration with masking cosmetics. Don't wear the perfume when
you are going to be in the sun. Keep it for use indoors or at
night.

Melasma (Mask of Pregnancy)

What causes the "mask of pregnancy"?

The mask of pregnancy refers to blotches of brownish pigmentation that may develop on the cheeks or forehead or around the
eyes of pregnant women and women who are taking birth control
pills. This problem is discussed in Chapter 7.

Freckles

Why do I freckle rather than tan when I go out in the sun?

You are undoubtedly a fair-skinned person who should avoid
deliberate sun exposure. You don't tan very well; instead, only
small, scattered groups of pigment-forming cells respond to the
sun's assault by forming freckles. Freckles are a warning to stay
out of the sun. If you do, your freckles will fade. When sun exposure is unavoidable, always use a sunscreen with a high SPF
(15 or more).

If your freckles are cosmetically troublesome, your demato-
logist may be able to treat them with a chemical peel or dermabrasion. They can also be minimized with makeup.

Senile Freckles

I never had freckles in my youth, but now that I'm getting older I have developed large freckles on the backs of my hands and my face and arms. What causes these spots? Is there any way to get rid of them?

The frecklelike brown spots that often appear on exposed areas of skin as a person ages may resemble the freckles of youth but they are larger and more irregular. Their color is darker and uneven, and they do not fade in winter. Although they are referred to as old-age or senile freckles, liver spots, or senile lentigines, there is no relationship between these spots and senility or liver disorders. They develop when the pigment-forming cells in some areas of the skin begin to produce too much pigment due to injury from years of sun exposure. The skin on these exposed areas also shows other signs of sun damage, such as premature aging.

By the time the brown spots appear, the skin has been irreversibly damaged. To help prevent the appearance of more senile freckles, you should protect the exposed skin areas by wearing an effective sunblock whenever you are outdoors. Nonetheless, some new lesions will inevitably develop because of the cumulative sun damage.

If the senile freckles change in any way—for example, if they become larger or thicker or develop a crust—you should consult a dermatologist. You may have a skin cancer that will require medical treatment.

Dermatologists can remove age spots with various techniques such as electrosurgery, freezing, and the application of certain chemicals.

Moles

What causes moles? Should they be removed?

The medical term for moles is *pigmented nevi*. They are distinct growths of various sizes and shapes and usually are brownish to brownish-black. The color is caused by the presence of special cells that contain melanin, the pigment responsible for skin color. Moles are rarely present at birth. Most appear during the first 20 years of life, but they may not appear until age 40 or later. Moles can appear anywhere on the skin, singly or in groups.

At first, moles are flat and brown or black, like freckles. With time, they usually enlarge and some may develop hairs. As the years advance, moles usually change slowly; most become elevated and lighter in color, although some will not change at all. Ultimately, most moles will slowly disappear; others may become raised, remaining connected to the skin by a small stalk. Sometimes the stalk becomes so slender that the moles fall off or are rubbed off. If the stalk twists, cutting off the blood supply, the mole may become swollen and darker and then drop off.

Moles may darken after exposure to the sun and sometimes during therapy with certain drugs. Moles also tend to become darker and larger during puberty and pregnancy.

If there are sudden changes in a mole's size, shape, or color, or if it bleeds, itches, or is painful, it is best to consult a dermatologist as soon as possible. What may appear to be a mole may actually be a skin cancer, such as a malignant melanoma.

Moles are frequently removed for cosmetic reasons. The most common methods of removal include superficial shave excision and excision with suture closure. Most such procedures take only a relatively short time and can be performed in a physician's office.

Moles and Skin Cancer

Do moles become cancerous?

Recent studies have shown that certain moles have a higher than average risk of becoming cancerous. Moles that are present at birth may fall into this group. The greatest risk is with those that are larger than 8 inches in diameter.

The presence of a special type of mole known as "dysplastic" may be a warning sign for the risk of developing skin cancer. These may be larger than the average mole (which is usually no larger than a pencil eraser) and more irregular. (It is said that those that are more than 0.6 centimeters in diameter are at greater risk of becoming cancerous.) They tend to be uneven in color, with dark brown centers and lighter edges. These moles tend to run in families, and it's estimated that about one in 25 Americans have them. Persons with this type of mole may be 10 times more likely to develop mole-related skin cancer than the average individual. If there is any question that the moles may be dysplastic, a dermatologist should be consulted.

You should also see a dermatologist if the appearance of a mole worries you or if it changes suddenly in any way. Moles that have the patriotic colors of red, white, and blue or contain black areas may have a greater chance of malignancy. You can obtain more information on moles from the American Academy of Dermatology.

Strawberry Birthmarks

What causes strawberry birthmarks? What treatment is recommended? Our baby has one on his shoulder.

"Strawberry mark" is the common name given to a vascular birthmark (hemangioma) that either is present at birth or appears during the first few months of life. It is elevated above the skin's surface, usually has a distinct border, and is red (thus resembling a strawberry), soft, and compressible. A strawberry mark can occur anywhere on the body. They are usually no larger than one or two inches in diameter; however, they can involve an entire limb.

Usually the lesion grows rapidly for the first several months, during which time it may increase several times in size. After a variable period, during which the size remains unchanged, the lesion begins to fade. As a rule, regression is very slow; two, four, or even six years may elapse before it disappears completely—but usually it is gone by the time the child is ready for school. Little, if any, cosmetic defect remains after spontaneous regression.

Reliable statistics show that there is complete spontaneous resolution of strawberry nevi in approximately 50% of patients by age five and in 70% by age seven. Even after that, continued improvement is common. Of the hemangiomas that do not regress, fewer than 10% are so cosmetically disturbing that they require treatment. For this reason, most dermatologists recommend waiting at least four years before considering treatment unless the hemangioma is causing a functional impairment (for instance, interfering with vision) or is subject to repeated bleeds. It is very difficult for parents to wait for the lesion to regress. It is even more difficult to watch the tumor enlarge without demanding that the physician do something.

Therapy for strawberry marks involves some risk, and the cosmetic results may not be as good as those produced by spontaneous regression. You should consult your physician about the pros and cons of treatment for your son's particular case. The physician will advise you of the various treatments that are available and recommend the most appropriate one if you decide to proceed with treatment rather than wait for regression.

You can write to the American Academy of Dermatology for more information about vascular birthmarks.

Port-Wine Stains

What causes the birthmark called a "port-wine stain"? What treatment is available?

Port-wine stains (nevus flammeus) are the most common type of vascular birthmark. Vascular birthmarks are caused by a congenital overgrowth of small blood vessels in the skin. A port-wine stain appears as a red, blue, or purplish discoloration of the skin. They are frequently seen on the face and neck; they are also common on the trunk, arms, and legs. The size can range from quite small to large enough to cover half of the face and body.

At birth, the surface of the port-wine stain is usually flat. Later in life, the birthmark may appear thicker and develop small bumps and ridges. If a port-wine stain appears on the back of the head or neck, or in an area normally covered by clothing, it may not be bothersome. Those on the face and throat or in other visible locations can cause considerable hardship.

Salmon-colored to red patches on the bridge of the nose and the back of the head in children usually disappear spontaneously. The few that might remain on the scalp are usually covered by hair. No treatment is indicated, but it is important to reassure the parents.

The emotional, social, and economic impact of these birthmarks should not be underestimated. They may significantly influence an individual's self-esteem, social interaction, and ability to gain certain types of employment.

In the past, most methods of treatment for the port-wine stain were less than satisfactory. The most practical one was to conceal the birthmark with special masking cosmetics. However, the advent of laser therapy has provided a satisfactory means of treating some port-wine stains.

You should consult your physician for referral to a recognized laser center for treatment. The American Academy of Dermatology can provide you with more information on port-wine stains.

Pityriasis Rosea

What is pityriasis rosea? It sounds dreadful.

The name is worse than the disorder. Pityriasis rosea is a com-

mon, benign, noncontagious skin rash of unknown cause. It produces few symptoms and most cases are mild. It can occur at any age but is more common in persons between the ages of 10 and 35 years.

The condition often begins with a single large, pink, usually scaly patch of skin on the chest or back. Called a "herald" or "mother" patch, it may be mistaken for a patch of ringworm, but unlike ringworm this disorder is not due to a fungus.

Within a week or two, many smaller pink patches will develop on the trunk and, to a lesser degree, over the arms and legs. Lesions may also occur on the neck, but rarely on the face.

The rash often develops into a characteristic pattern over the back, resembling the outline of an evergreen tree with drooping branches. Sometimes the skin reaction is more severe, with more irritation. On rare occasions, itching can be quite severe, particularly when the individual becomes overheated.

The rash usually fades and disappears within six weeks after peak activity but can sometimes last much longer. It heals without scarring. Various environmental or physical factors can cause transient worsening or even reappearance of the rash. These include physical exertion, such as running, or bathing in hot water.

Diagnosis of pityriasis rosea can be made by a dermatologist. Treatment may include external and internal medications to relieve the itching, although this is rarely necessary. If pityriasis appears before a special occasion, such as a wedding or prom, when a lowcut gown would reveal the skin problem, systemic steroids will clear up the rash. You can obtain more information on pityriasis rosea from the American Academy of Dermatology.

Tinea Versicolor

What is tinea versicolor? How does it affect the pigment of the skin?

Tinea versicolor is a superficial infection of the upper layers of the skin. To the patient, the major concern is the uneven skin pigmentation and scaly areas, presenting a cosmetic problem.

The infection is caused by a yeastlike fungus that normally lives on the skin surface in small numbers. The fungus thrives best in oily areas of the skin, such as the neck, upper chest, and back. Under conditions of increased heat, humidity, and sweating, the fungus proliferates and can then invade the outer layer of skin.

The infection is usually seen as small and slowly enlarging scaly, white-to-tan spots scattered over the upper arms, chest, and back. Sometimes the spots appear on the neck and face. On light skin the spots may not be noticeable or they may show up as tan-to-pink spots.

Tinea versicolor may first become obvious when the skin becomes tanned because the fungus, either by producing a substance or by acting as a physical shield, prevents the involved areas from tanning. The involved skin may also peel, leaving the skin lighter in color. On dark skin, the lesions are very noticeable. They appear as discrete spots that are white to pale tan and have a slightly scaly surface. Aside from the changes in pigmentation, tinea versicolor produces few symptoms except occasional itching.

Teenagers and young adults are most susceptible to tinea versicolor infections. It is very rare in the elderly and uncommon in children, except in tropical climates. People with oily skin seem to be more susceptible to infection than those with dry skin. The rash is easily diagnosed and treated. Recurrences are quite common, especially when conditions favor growth of the fungus. Your dermatologist may choose from various topical and oral medications. However, the cosmetic defect of uneven pigmentation of the skin remains for many months after the fungus has been eliminated.

More information on tinea versicolor is available by writing to the American Academy of Dermatology.

26

The Skin and AIDS

Skin Conditions Associated with AIDS

What are the skin conditions associated with AIDS? Are they unique to AIDS patients?

A number of skin conditions, particularly infections, have been seen in association with AIDS (acquired immunodeficiency syndrome) and infection with HIV (human immunodeficiency virus). Sometimes the first clue to an HIV infection is a skin disorder. One of the most widely publicized of these is a rare form of Kaposi's sarcoma (see the following question and answer). A condition that involves the tongue, known as oral "hairy" leukoplakia, has so far been found only in patients infected with HIV.

Other skin conditions found in patients with AIDS also occur in patients without AIDS. *Therefore, it must be emphasized that since most of the skin eruptions seen in AIDS patients are also seen in other patients, their presence does not necessarily indicate that the patient has an HIV infection.* However, in HIV-infected patients the skin conditions are frequently more severe and often more difficult to treat. These other common skin conditions include viral infections such as herpes simplex, herpes zoster ("shingles"), warts, molluscum contagiosum, fungal infections such as oral candidiasis ("thrush"), bacterial infections such as impetigo, psoriasis, and seborrheic dermatitis.

If any of these skin problems occurs in an individual who thinks that he or she may be at high risk for AIDS and the problem is very severe, recurrent, or unresponsive to treatment, the individual should seek the advice of a dermatologist for evaluation, diagnosis, and treatment. It should be stressed again that these problems are also common in healthy individuals. Detailed discussions of most of these skin conditions are found in the following answers.

Kaposi's Sarcoma

What is Kaposi's sarcoma? I understand that it is very common in AIDS.

One type of Kaposi's sarcoma, a very rare form of cancer, is a very common skin manifestation of AIDS. About 20% of AIDS patients develop Kaposi's sarcoma. The dermatologist is often the first physician to make the diagnosis of Kaposi's sarcoma, usually by performing a small tissue biopsy in the office or clinic.

The lesions of Kaposi's sarcoma do not hurt or itch. They can appear anywhere on the skin or in the mouth (especially on the front part of the palate and on the gums). The lesions vary in color from pink to dark red, purple, or brown, and are often mistaken for insect bites, birthmarks, or bruises. The lesions range from the size of a pinhead to that of a large coin, and frequently continue to develop into firm bumps and even large tumor growths. They may be single or multiple lesions, with new ones developing anyplace on the skin during the course of the illness. Occasionally Kaposi's sarcoma can involve the lymph nodes, as well as internal organs such as the spleen, liver, stomach or bowel, and the lungs.

Large, individual tumors, such as those located on the face or other exposed areas, can be treated with local X-ray therapy or even surgically removed by a dermatologist. In patients with widespread disease, chemotherapy may be given under the supervision of a physician.

It should be emphasized that another type of Kaposi's sarcoma can be seen without AIDS.

Viral Skin Infections and AIDS

Please discuss the common viral infections associated with AIDS.

Viral infections of the skin are very common in patients with AIDS. These infections can occur on the skin or mucous membrane (for example, in the mouth, eyes, nose, and rectal and genital areas). In AIDS patients these viral infections are sometimes more severe than in healthy individuals.

The *herpes simplex* virus is responsible for the recurrent infections commonly called "fever blisters" or "cold sores" that appear around the nose and mouth. Repeated herpes infections also occur in the eyes and in the anal and genital regions, but any area of the skin can be involved. The first indication of a lesion may be a sensation of burning, itching, tingling, or pain. Before the blisters or ulcers develop, the involved area usually becomes red. The clusters of tiny blisters break, leaving small erosions or ulcers which may develop crusts. Herpes infections usually heal within five to 10 days. Patients infected with HIV who develop herpes tend to experience more severe outbreaks with large, painful ulcerations that often increase in size, lasting for three to four weeks or longer, instead of quickly healing in 5–10 days as occurs in non-HIV-infected individuals.

Dermatologists and other physicians may prescribe a specific oral antiviral medication for these severe outbreaks of herpes. Topical medications are also used, to dry up the lesions and relieve discomfort. Antibiotics may be recommended if the lesions become further infected with bacteria. In immune-suppressed patients, herpes infections can spread widely within the body, with the development of symptoms such as high fever, mental confusion, headaches, and weakness. Hospitalization may be necessary.

The *herpes zoster* virus is responsible for the skin infection commonly referred to as "shingles," which may be the first sign that a patient has been infected with HIV and has a weakened immune system. The same virus that causes chicken pox in childhood, it may remain dormant in the body until reactivated as shingles. The eruption appears suddenly in a bandlike pattern limited to an area of the skin on one side of the body. The involved area becomes tender and red, and there may be deep, throbbing pain. Clusters of fragile blisters appear, and leave ulcers after they rupture. The severe pain that is typical of herpes zoster is due to inflammation of the nerves in the involved region. The condition can last for several weeks and occasionally spreads to other parts of the body, with blisters developing that look like chicken pox.

Topical lotions and oral antiviral medications may be useful in drying up the blisters and ulcers. The pain, which may be severe, can sometimes be relieved with special medications prescribed by a physician. For patients who develop severe or widespread herpes zoster, hospitalization may be necessary so that intravenous antiviral medication can be administered.

Oral "hairy" leukoplakia is an unusual condition characterized by small, white, fuzzy patches that are most often seen on the tongue. This condition has only recently been described and has so far been observed only in HIV-infected individuals. Hairy leukoplakia is believed to be caused by a member of the herpes family known as the Epstein-Barr virus. It can be confused with "thrush," a yeast infection of the mouth, which is also commonly seen in individuals infected with HIV. There are no symptoms associated with hairy leukoplakia. The development of this condition is not known to cause any problems, but it is an important signal to the patient and physician that the patient is probably infected with HIV.

Other viral disorders, including warts and molluscum contagiosum, may be common and more severe in patients with AIDS. See Chapter 19 for more information on these diseases.

Yeast Infections and AIDS

I would appreciate information on yeast infections such as thrush when associated with AIDS.

Yeast infections involving the mouth, the vagina, the skin folds under the arms, and the groin region caused by *Candida albicans* (*Monilia*) frequently and repeatedly occur in many patients with AIDS. When such yeast infections develop in the mouth, they are commonly known as "thrush." Thrush appears as white, curdlike patches that are easily scraped off. The patches occur on the tongue and inner surfaces of the cheeks. Thrush can be easily confused with hairy leukoplakia, described in the previous answer. It commonly causes soreness of the mouth or throat, difficulty in swallowing, and loss of taste. The infection can also spread from the throat into the gastrointestinal tract, causing a burning sensation in the chest upon swallowing.

Both adults and infants who have HIV infection and AIDS frequently develop yeast infections of the skin characterized by a severe itchy red rash involving the skin folds, such as the groin and under the breasts in women. These infections may be treated by a dermatologist with topical creams and orally administered drugs. However, in patients infected with HIV, yeast infections are sometimes resistant to traditional treatment and often reappear after treatment is stopped. Women with AIDS may develop severe, treatment-resistant vaginitis due to *Candida* infections, characterized by a milky white vaginal discharge. Dermatologists may prescribe local topical preparations or oral medications for vaginal candidiasis.

Bacterial Infections and AIDS

What are the common bacterial skin infections associated with AIDS?

Patients infected with HIV frequently develop a variety of bacterial skin infections. Intravenous drug abusers may develop abscesses at the injection sites. The bacterial infection most commonly seen in HIV-infected patients is impetigo, characterized by the widespread development of multiple clusters of large, soft, fluid-filled blisters that tend to break easily, oozing yellowish liquid (see Chapter 20). Once the blisters break, flat reddish areas remain.

In AIDS patients, there is the danger that these bacterial infections can spread into the bloodstream. Therefore, intravenous antibiotic therapy may be indicated.

Other Common Skin Disorders Aggravated in AIDS Patients

Are common disorders such as seborrheic dermatitis and psoriasis aggravated in AIDS patients?

Yes, seborrheic dermatitis, psoriasis, and some other common skin disorders, including hives and folliculitis, are much worse in AIDS patients, and more resistant to treatment. However, treatment measures are the same as when the disorders occur in other individuals. For complete details about these disorders, see the discussions of seborrheic dermatitis in Chapters 2 and 7 and psoriasis in Chapter 23.

27

Skin Cancer

Solar Keratoses

What are solar keratoses? Should they be removed?

Solar (actinic) keratoses are precancerous skin growths. They vary greatly in appearance but usually appear as red, scaly, rough areas of varying sizes on sun-exposed skin. As the name indicates, they are caused by overexposure to the sun.

Some of these lesions may develop into squamous cell carcinomas and therefore should be treated. Freezing with liquid nitrogen and electrosurgery are two common treatment methods. If the lesions are extensive, a chemical (5-fluorouracil) may be used.

To prevent the development of solar keratoses later in life, avoid overexposure to the sun and protect the skin with clothing and effective sunblocks when sun exposure is unavoidable.

Basal Cell and Squamous Cell Skin Cancers

What are the differences between basal cell and squamous cell skin cancers? How are they treated?

Basal cell carcinoma (cancer) is the most common form of skin cancer, affecting over 400,000 Americans per year. People with fair skin and blue or green eyes are most susceptible to this form of skin cancer. As the name indicates, basal cell cancers develop from the basal cells that lie at the base of the epidermis, the outer layer of skin. The clinical manifestations vary greatly but a basal cell carcinoma usually appears as a small, shiny, fleshy nodule with a central depression. They are very slow-growing and often take many months or years to reach a diameter of ½ to one inch. Untreated, a basal cancer will alternately bleed and crust over. In fact, any sore, especially on sun-exposed areas, that keeps crusting over and doesn't heal should be considered a potential basal cell carcinoma. The most common sites for these lesions are the face, the top of bald heads, the neck, and the upper back and chest—areas subject to sun exposure.

This type of cancer rarely, if ever, metastasizes (spreads) to other parts of the body, but it can extend below the skin, even to the underlying bone, causing considerable tissue destruction. As the lesions enlarge, they outgrow their blood supply, resulting in ulceration.

Squamous cell carcinoma, the next most common form of skin cancer, affects over 100,000 people per year in the United States. These lesions, which arise from squamous cells in the upper part of the epidermis, usually appear as red, scaly patches or pinkish opaque lumps with or without central ulcers. Squamous cell carcinomas will increase in size, frequently developing into large, raised tumors. In contrast to basal cell carcinomas, squamous cell carcinomas can metastasize, although this is rare when they occur on sun-damaged skin. These cancers are most common on the rim of the ear, the face, and the lips and mouth.

Both forms of skin cancer are rare in dark-skinned individuals. Those with a light complexion, blue eyes, and light hair are most susceptible. These are the same individuals who are most susceptible to damage from sun exposure.

Fortunately, both forms of cancer are relatively easy to treat, especially if treatment is initiated early. The cure rate is 95%. There are several methods of treatment, including surgical removal, curettage and electrosurgery, Mohs micrographic (microscopically controlled) surgery, x-ray therapy, freezing (cryosurgery), and laser therapy. Treatment depends on the type, location, and size of the lesion, and the patient's medical history.

If you develop any type of growth that changes color, increases in diameter, becomes elevated, acquires an irregular border, becomes sensitive or hurts, becomes crusted, bleeds easily, or does not heal, consult a dermatologist for diagnosis and treatment. The dermatologist may be able to determine whether the growth is benign, precancerous, or malignant just by inspection. However, to confirm or establish the diagnosis, the dermatologist may remove a portion of the tissue and submit it for microscopic examination (a biopsy).

You can obtain detailed information on skin cancers from the American Academy of Dermatology.

Beware of Malignant Melanoma

Why is malignant melanoma so serious? I thought all skin cancers were relatively harmless and curable. How do you tell it apart from other kinds of skin cancer?

While most skin cancers are relatively easily treated (see previous answer), malignant melanoma is different. It has a greater potential to metastasize (spread) to other parts of the body, and it may be fatal. But melanoma is almost always curable in its early stages.

Malignant melanoma involves the pigment-forming cells of the skin and appears as a dark brown or black growth with irregular borders and irregular pigmentation. Certain nevi (moles) have an increased risk for the development of melanoma. These include special types of nevi, called dysplastic nevi, which have an irregular shape and uneven coloration. These moles may be single or multiple and may or may not run in families. People with more than average (over 40) nevi, especially when they vary widely in size, shape, and color, are also in the higher-risk group.

The most frequent sites for melanoma are the upper back of both men and women, the anterior torso of men, and the lower legs of women. Melanomas are relatively rare in dark-skinned individuals, but when they do occur in non-white races, the site is usually the palms, soles, or mucous membranes.

Although the incidence of melanoma is relatively low in comparison to that of other forms of skin cancer, it is rapidly rising. Dermatologists are seeing almost twice as many melanomas today as they saw 20 years ago. Melanoma currently strikes over 27,000 people a year and is fatal to over 7,000 patients a year. Experts believe that this increased incidence is possibly due in part to our love affair with the sun. But it doesn't require chronic overexposure to the sun to predispose an individual to melanoma: Researchers have shown that one severe, blistering sunburn during childhood or adolescence makes an individual twice as likely to develop malignant melanoma later in life. Heredity also plays a role in malignant melanoma. If your parents, children, or siblings have had a melanoma, your risk of developing one is increased 8 to 12 times.

Age, skin type, and history of previous melanomas are important factors too. Melanoma is an adult disease. The incidence at age 15 or older is 40 times greater than at 14 or younger. Individuals with fair skin that sunburns easily and tans poorly, or those with light hair, blue or hazel eyes, or freckles are at two to seven times greater risk because they are more susceptible to sun damage. If you have already had one melanoma, your chances are 900 times greater that you will develop another one, usually within three years. However, the end of the third year is not a cutoff point, and you should continue to have regular skin checks at least once a year.

Since early detection and treatment is the key to surviving malignant melanoma, you should be alert to any changes in pigmented lesions—in color, shape, size, or thickness. The Academy of Dermatology recommends the "ABCD guideline":

Asymmetry: a lopsided shape.
Border: irregular edges that are ragged, notched, or blurred.
Color: pigmentation that is not uniform; shades of tan, brown, and black are present. Dashes of red, white, and blue add to the mottled appearance.
Diameter: growth to the size of a pencil eraser or larger.

Consult a dermatologist immediately if you notice any of these changes.

To minimize your chances of developing malignant melanoma, you should practice sensible habits for protection from the sun, since skin specialists believe that acute sunburning is an important factor accounting for the increase in the rate of melanomas. If we do not change our habit of sun worship, it is predicted that about one of every 100 people born in the year 2000 will develop a melanoma during his or her lifetime. Next to lung cancer, it is the fastest rising malignancy in women. Many factors, including a longer lifespan, depletion of the ozone layer, and increased outdoor recreation time probably have contributed to the increase in skin cancers.

Kaposi's Sarcoma

What is Kaposi's sarcoma? I've heard so much about it recently.

Kaposi's sarcoma is a tumor of the blood vessels that previously was considered very rare and was seen primarily in elderly men. More recently, a variation of Kaposi's sarcoma has been seen in patients with acquired immunodeficiency syndrome (AIDS).

Kaposi's sarcoma in AIDS is probably the same disease as that seen previously, but the manifestations are different in the immune-depressed patient. Most of the lesions are flat, stainlike, and insignificant, testing the physician's diagnostic ability. The association of other risk factors (homosexuality, intravenous drug use, hemophilia) and clinical findings such as weight loss, loss of vigor, and recurring infectious disease (*Pneumocystis carinii*, viral diseases, deep fungus infections) help establish the clinical diagnosis of AIDS. Once AIDS is diagnosed, the diagnosis of Kaposi's sarcoma is easier. (See Chapter 26 for more information on AIDS.)

Skin Cancer and the Sun

Is it true one of the primary causes of skin cancer is overexposure to the sun?

The principal cause of skin cancer is almost universally accepted by medical experts to be overexposure to sunlight, especially when it results in sunburn and blistering. Ninety percent of all skin cancers occur on parts of the body that are unprotected by clothing. The only exception is melanoma, which may appear on areas never exposed to the sun.

Farmers and others who work outdoors, sports enthusiasts, sun-worshippers, and everyone else who by choice or necessity spends many hours in the sun are likely candidates for leathery complexions and solar keratoses (precancerous growths).

Those individuals whose fair skin and light eyes and hair make them most susceptible to sunburn and other sun damage are also at higher risk for developing skin cancer. Skin cancer is less common in blacks, whose pigmentation acts as a natural sunblock.

The incidence of skin cancer also tends to be higher in areas of the country where the intensity of sunlight is highest—the South and Southwest.

Those who drive with the window open expose the left side of their faces to the sun; in the United States skin cancers are more prevalent on that side. In England and Australia, where drivers sit on the right side of their cars, cancer is more common on the right side of the face.

Unlike sun worshippers who feel that bronzed skin is a sign of health and vitality, dermatologists view tanning as a response to injury. Evidence indicates that the sun's ultraviolet rays kill some skin cells on contact and injure others. Over a long period of time, overexposure to these rays can leave the skin mottled with brown spots intermingled with yellowish areas. Eventually, skin cancers may appear.

Of course, other factors may also cause skin cancer, although they are much less common. These include excessive medical and industrial x-ray exposure, scarring from burns, and occupational exposure to such compounds as tar and arsenic. Genetic factors may also play a role in one's susceptibility to skin cancers, especially in certain melanomas (see the question and answer on melanomas elsewhere in this chapter).

The skin can be protected from the sun with protective clothing and sunscreens with a high SPF rating. For more details on sunscreens, see Chapter 21.

Self-Exam for Skin Cancer

Do you recommend regular self-examination for skin cancer?

Absolutely. Prevention and early detection of melanomas and other skin cancers are obviously the most desirable weapons against these cancers. To help ensure that any developing lesion is caught in the early stage, dermatologists recommend that you institute a regular program of monthly self-examination. Get familiar with your skin and your own pattern of moles, freckles, and "beauty marks." Be alert to changes in the number, size, shape, and color of pigmented areas. If you notice any changes, see your dermatologist. When lesions are caught in the early stages they are almost always totally curable.

The following is a suggested method of self-examination that will ensure that no area of the body is neglected.

1. You will need a full-length mirror, a hand mirror, and a brightly lit room where you can study your skin in privacy.
2. Examine your body, front and back, in the mirror. Then examine the right and left sides, with arms raised.
3. Bend your elbows and look carefully at your forearms and upper underarms and palms.
4. Next, look at the backs of the legs and the feet, including the soles and between the toes.
5. Examine the back of the neck and the scalp with the help of a hand mirror; part your hair (or use a blow dryer) to give you a close look.
6. Finally, check your back and buttocks with a hand mirror.

If you cannot see areas using this method, have them looked at by a family member or friend. If you have any suspicious lesions, see your dermatologist.

Index

Hair waving/straightening (*contd.*)
  precautions/limitations for
    chemical straighteners, 59-60
    techniques for, 55-56
  wave-setting preparations, 54-55
Hair weaving, 23
Hands:
  eczema on, 165-166
  fissures on palms and fingers, 168
  "housewife's dermatitis," 164-165
  "liver spots," 166-167
  sweaty palms, 167-168
    controlling, 185-186
Hangnails, 171-172
"Hard top" hairpieces, 22
Hard water for bathing, soft water
    versus, 154
Head lice, 205-206
Heat and humidity:
  acne and, 267
  effect on the skin of, 217
Heels, rough skin on, 158-159
Hemorrhages on the feet (from
    sports), 235
Henna, 39
Herb baths, 154
Heredity, acne and, 267
Herpes infections, 281-287
  in babies, 284-285
  chicken pox, 281, 287
  cold sores, 281-282, 299, 301
  fever blisters, 281-282, 301
  genital herpes, 283-284
    sexual exposure and, 284
  shingles, 281, 286-287, 301
Herpes simplex, 281-282, 299, 301
Herpes zoster, 281, 286-287, 299,
    301
Hirsutism, *see* Excess hair
Hives, 190-191
Home electrolysis devices, 143-144
Homemade facial products, 105-106
Home permanents, professional
    permanents versus, 50
Hormone creams, 98-99
Hormones:
  acne and, 263-264
  excessive hair growth and, 134
Hot aerosol shaving creams, 126

"Hot pressing" for straightening
    hair, 56-57
Hot water, dry skin and, 153-154
"Housewife's dermatitis," 164-165
Humidity and heat:
  acne and, 267
  effect on the skin of, 217
Hyaluronic acid in creams and
    lotions, 101-102
Hyperpigmentation:
  from acne, 265
  of black skin, 291
  from perfume, 291-292

Icepick-type acne scars, treatment
    for, 271-272
Ichthyosis, very dry skin versus,
    148-149
Impetigo, 299
Infant skin care, 214-215
Infections around the nails, 174
Infrared radiation (IR), 239
Ingrown beard hairs, 129-130
Ingrown toenails, 178-179
Insect repellents, 202-203
Insects and bugs, 201-208
  bedbugs, 204-205
  bees, 201-202
  chiggers, 202
  crabs, 205
  creeping eruptions, 208
  fleas, 208
  head lice, 205-206
  mosquitoes, 202-203
  sand flies, 207
  scabies, 206-207
  spiders, 203-204
  wasps, 201-202
Inverse psoriasis, 274
Iron deficiency anemia, hair loss
    due to, 15
Irritations:
  allergies versus, 189-190
  from football pads, 233
  from helmet chinstraps, 233

Jewelry, allergic reactions to,
    191-192
Jock itch, 234

Jogger's nipples, 232-233
Jogging shoes, blisters from,
   235-236

Kaposi's sarcoma (KS), 309
  AIDS and, 300

Lanolin, allergic reactions to,
   194-195
Lead acetate dyes, 33, 38
Legal problems with anti-aging
   creams, 106-107
Leg hair:
  removing, 151
  shaving, 152
Legs, telangiectasia and varicosities
   of, 218
Lentigines, see Age spots
Lightening dark complexions, 81
Light permanent waves, 48-49
Liposomes in cosmetic creams,
   100-101
Liposuction:
  for aging skin, 118-119
  for excess fat, 152-153
Lips, chapped, 82
Liquid facial "soaps," 73
Lithium, acne and, 268-269
"Liver spots" on the hands, 166-167
Lubricating creams, 94-96
Lupus erythematosus, 248

Makeup, see Facial products
Male-pattern baldness (MPB), 17-18
Malignant melanoma, 307-308
Mascara for contact lens wearers,
  89
Masking birthmarks, makeup for,
   80-81
Massage for aging skin, 121-122
Medicated soaps, 73
  for acne, 262
Medications as cause of excess hair,
   134-135
Medulla, 3
Melanin (pigment), 5
Melanocytes, 6
Melanoma, malignant, 307-308
Melasma (mask of pregnancy),

83-84, 292
  bleaching creams for, 104-105
Men, hair dyes for, 41
Menopause, excess facial hair after,
  135
Metal jewelry, allergic reactions to,
   191-192
Microcirculation, creams to
  improve, 98
Milia, 82-83
Milk baths, 154
Mineral oil in creams, 102
Minoxidil, 18-19
Mist rollers, 53
Moisturizers:
  petroleum jelly as, 103
  phospholipids in, 97
Moisturizing creams, 94-96
  application of, 96
Moles (pigmented nevi), 293-294
  skin cancer and, 294
Molluscum, 299
Mosquitoes, 202-203
Mousses, 55, 69-70
Mucopolysaccharides in creams
  and lotions, 101-102

Nails, 169-179
  brittle nails, 173
  discoloration of, 175-176
  grooves in, 172
  hangnails, 171-172
  hardeners, 176
  infections of the cuticles and
   skin around, 174
  nail tips, 178
  press-on, 177
  "sculptured" acrylic, 176-177
  separation of, 174-175
  skin disorders and, 171
  structure of, 169-171
  toenails, ingrown, 178-179
  white spots on, 172-173
  wrapping, 177-178
Natural-bristle hair brushes, 9
Natural cosmetics, 106
Natural moisturizing factor (NMF),
  96-97
Newborn acne, 269

Nickel, allergic reactions to, 191-192
Normal hair loss, 11
Nose, rhinophyma of, 86
Nylon hair brushes, 9

Oily foods, 210
Oily hair, 29-30
    shampooing, 3
Oily skin:
    care of, 75
    shaving creams for, 127
    soap for, 73
    the summer and, 75-76
Oral candidiasis, 299
Oral contraceptives, hair loss and,
    14
Oral "hairy" leukoplakia, 299, 302
Oral retinoids for severe acne,
    259-260
Oxygen, aging skin and, 116

Painting (hair painting), 44-45
Palmar warts, 225
Palms:
    fissures on, 168
    sweaty, 167-168
        controlling, 185-186
Para-aminobenzoic acid (PABA),
    196
Paraphenylenediamine (PPD), 196
Partial hairpieces, 22
Patch tests, 37, 39-40
Peel-off facial masks, 79
Perfume, hyperpigmentation from
    291-292
Perianal warts, 226
Permanent eyeliners, 90-91
Permanent oxidation dyes, 33, 36-38
Permanent waving, see Hair
    waving/straightening
Perspiration:
    antiperspirants, 182, 183-184
    body odor and, 181-182
    controlling sweaty palms, 185-186
    deodorant soaps, 184-185
    deodorants, 183-184
    excessive, 182-183
        surgery for, 183
    prickly heat, 145-146, 188

yellow staining of clothes due to,
    187-188
Persulfate boosters, 46
    reactions to, 45-46
Petechiae from exercise, 234
Petroleum jelly as a moisturizer,
    103
pH of skin-care products, 224
Phospholipids in creams, 97
Photosensitivity of the skin, 248-249
Pigtails, hair loss from, 13
Pill, the, hair loss and, 14
Pityriasis rosea, 296-297
Plantar warts, 225
Plucking, removing excess hair by,
    139-140
Poison ivy dermatitis, 196-198
Pomades for straightening hair, 56
Pores:
    closing of, 219
    enlarged, 83
Prophyria cutanea tarda, 248
Port-wine stains (birthmarks), 296
Pregnancy:
    hair loss and, 13-14
    melasma during, 83-84, 292
        bleaching creams for, 104-105
    permanent waving and, 51
    skin care during, 213-214
Preservatives in cosmetics, allergic
    reactions to, 192-193
Preshave preparation, 124-125
Press-on nails, 177
Prickly heat (miliaria), 145-146, 188
Professional permanents, home
    permanents versus, 50
Protein deficiencies affecting the
    skin and hair, 211
Psoriasis, 273-279, 299, 303
    forms of, 274-275
    as incurable, 276
    scalp psoriasis, 276-277
    therapy for, 275-276
    coal tar, 277
    etretinate, 278-279
    PUVA, 277-278
Pumice stone for removal of excess
    facial hair, 140
PUVA (psoralen plus UVA light), 277-278

Rashes, 189
  caused by reactions to food, 220
  caused by reactions to jewelry
    and other metals, 191-192
  diaper, 215-216
Redheads, 6
Red neck from sun exposure, 251
Red spots, *see* Cayenne pepper
  spots
Resorcin, 261
Retinoic acid for aging skin,
  120-121
Retinoids for acne, 258-260
Rhinophyma, 86
Rosacea, 85
Rough skin on the heels, 158-159
Rubber gloves for prevention of
  "housewife's dermatitis," 165
Rubber products, allergic reactions
  to, 195

Salicylic acid, 261
Sand flies, 207
Scabies, 206-207
Scalp psoriasis, 276-277
Scalp-reduction surgery, 21
Scars:
  recommended treatment for,
    216-217
  See also Acne, scars from
"Sculptured" acrylic nails, 176-177
Seborrheic dermatitis, 25-26, 84-85,
  299, 303
Seborrheic keratoses, 211-222
Self-examination for skin cancer,
  310-311
Semi-permanent hair-coloring
  preparations, 33, 35-36
Senile freckles, 292-293
Separation of nails, 174-175
Sexual activity:
  acne and, 268
  genital herpes and, 284
Shampoos, 61-63
  for dandruff treatment, 26
  dry (waterless), 64
  frequency of, 3-4, 8
  soap as, 63-64
  special additives in, 63

Shaving, 123-131
  acne and, 131, 264
  aftershave preparations, 127
  barber's itch, 129
  beards
    heavy, dark beards, 128
    ingrown hairs, 129-130
    preparation before wet shaving,
      125
    problems under beards, 128
  blacks and ingrown beard hairs,
    130
  creams for oily or dry skins, 127
  electric versus blade shaving,
    123-124
  the legs and underarms, 151, 152
  preparations for, 125-127
  preshave preparations, 124-125
  removing excess facial hair,
    136-137
  warts and, 130-131
Shingles (herpes zoster), 281,
  286-287, 299, 301
Shoe leather, allergic reactions to,
  193-194
Singeing the hair, 31-32
Skiing, sun protection while,
  247-248
Skin cancer, 305-311
  basal cell carcinoma, 305-307
  Kaposi's sarcoma, 309
  malignant melanoma, 307-308
  moles and, 294
  self-examination for, 310-311
  solar keratoses, 250, 305
  squamos cell carcinoma, 305-307
  sun and, 309-310
Skin's natural moisturizing factor
  (NMF), 96-97
Slow cell turnover, aging skin due
  to, 112-113
Soap(s):
  allergic reactions to, 193
  cleansing the face with, 72-73, 94
  creams and lotions versus soap
    and water, 94
  deodorant, 184-185
  irritation caused by, 189-190
  for shampooing, 63-64

Soap(s) (contd.)
for shaving, 125, 126
Soft corns, 162
"Soft mat" hair pieces, 22
Soft water for bathing, hard water
versus, 154
Solar (actinic) keratoses, 250, 305
Soles of the feet, fissures on, 168
SPF (sun protection factor) on
sunscreens, 240-241
Spider bites, 203-204
Split ends, cure for, 31
Sports-related skin problems,
229-237
abrasions, 236
acne and irritation from helmet
chinstraps, 233
athlete's foot, 162-163, 236-237
treatment of, 163-164
blisters, 235-236
buttocks acne and folliculitis, 231
exercise machines and acne, 231
hemorrhages on the feet, 235
irritation from football pads, 233
jock itch, 234
jogger's nipples, 232-233
petechiae from exercise, 234
swimmer's ear, 229-230
swimmer's skin and hair, 230
weightlifting and stretch marks,
232
wrestling and skin infections, 223
Squamous cell carcinoma, 305-307
Staining of clothes due to
perspiration, 187-188
Steroid (corticosteroid) acne, 270
Straightening hair, see Hair waving
and straightening
Straight hair, curly hair versus, 5-6
Strawberry birthmarks, 295
Streaking hair, 44-45
Stretch garments, allergic reactions
to, 195
Stretch marks, 146
caused by weightlifting, 232
Sulfur in acne medications, 261
Summer, care of oily skin during,
75-76
Sun and skin, 239-251

aging skin care, 113
fake tans, 245-246
photosensitivity of the skin,
248-249
protection for children, 244-245
protective clothing, 244
red neck due to exposure, 251
skiing and, 247-248
skin cancer, 309-310
solar (actinic) keratoses, 250, 305
tanning
dangers of, 239-240, 242-243
tips on, 243
tanning accelerators, 246-247
umbrellas, 244
water sports and, 251
white spots on tanned skin, 250
working in the sun, 240
Sunburns, treatment for, 246
Sun poisoning, 249-251
Sun-related diseases, 248
Sunscreens:
for hair, 4, 69
ingredients in, 241-242
SPF number on, 240-241
Suntan parlors, dangers of, 247
Superfatted soaps, 73
Superficial chemosurgery for aging
skin, 119-120
Surgery for excessive perspiration,
183
Sweaty, smelly feet, 159-160
Sweaty palms, 167-168
controlling, 185-186
Swimming:
hair and skin problems caused
by, 30-31, 230
swimmer's ear, 229-230

Tanning:
dangers of, 239-240, 242-243
tips on, 243
Tanning accelerators, 246-247
Tar and acne, 269
Tattoo removal, 223-224
Telangiectasia of the legs, 218
Temporary hair-coloring products,
33, 34-35
Thioglycolate hair straighteners, 58